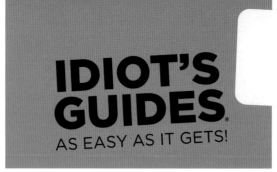
IDIOT'S GUIDES.
AS EASY AS IT GETS!

Autoimmune Cookbook

by Amari Thomsen, MS, RD, LDN

ALPHA

A member of Penguin Random House LLC

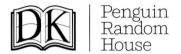

Publisher: Mike Sanders
Associate Publisher: Billy Fields
Acquisitions Editor: Nathalie Mornu
Cover and Book Designer: William Thomas
Development Editor: Ann Barton
Compositor: Ayanna Lacey
Proofreader: Amy Borrelli
Indexer: Heather McNeill

First American Edition, 2015
Published in the United States by DK Publishing
6081 E. 82nd Street, Indianapolis, Indiana 46250

A Penguin Random House Company

19   10 9 8 7 6 5

005–285183–December2015

Published in the United States by Dorling Kindersley Limited.

ISBN: 978-1-61564-866-5

Library of Congress Catalog Card Number: 2015942375

Printed in China

Note: This publication contains the opinions and ideas of its author(s). It is intended to provide helpful and informative material on the subject matter covered. It is sold with the understanding that the author(s) and publisher are not engaged in rendering professional services in the book. If the reader requires personal assistance or advice, a competent professional should be consulted. The author(s) and publisher specifically disclaim any responsibility for any liability, loss, or risk, personal or otherwise, which is incurred as a consequence, directly or indirectly, of the use and application of any of the contents of this book.

Trademarks: All terms mentioned in this book that are known to be or are suspected of being trademarks or service marks have been appropriately capitalized. Alpha Books, DK, and Penguin Random House LLC cannot attest to the accuracy of this information. Use of a term in this book should not be regarded as affecting the validity of any trademark or service mark.

DK books are available at special discounts when purchased in bulk for sales promotions, premiums, fund-raising, or educational use. For details, contact: DK Publishing Special Markets, 345 Hudson Street, New York, New York 10014 or SpecialSales@dk.com.

www.dk.com

A WORLD OF IDEAS
SEE ALL THERE IS TO KNOW

Contents

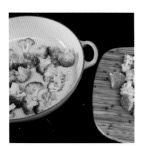 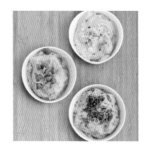 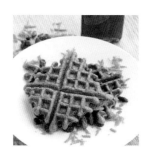 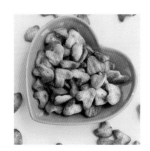

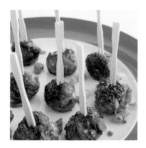
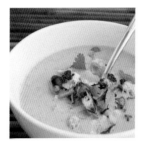
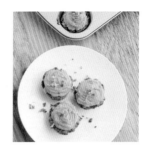
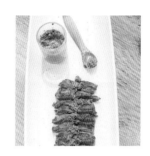

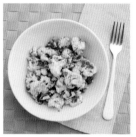 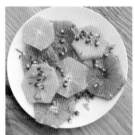 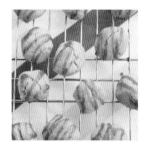 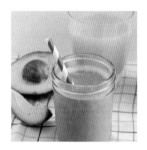

Introduction

An autoimmune disease refers to an illness characterized by a misguided immune system, which causes an attack on the body's own healthy tissues.

A common attribute of an autoimmune disorder is inflammation of the gastrointestinal system. The autoimmune protocol (AIP) diet encourages the consumption of foods that decrease inflammation, heal the gut, and assist in the restoration of healthy immune system function.

Having worked with clients with autoimmune conditions and digestive disorders, I can appreciate and understand the challenges that come along with adopting such a unique new diet. Many fear the idea of avoiding the foods they are most familiar with. Understanding which foods to avoid and adjusting to a new way of cooking can seem daunting at first. But take it upon yourself to channel positive creativity and curiosity. Find excitement in trying new things and experimenting with alternative ingredients. Embrace the power that comes along with being conscious of the foods you put in your body and how they make you feel.

The recipes in this book are designed to help you transition into your new AIP lifestyle without feeling deprived. In addition to delicious recipes, you will find tips and tricks to help you along the way as well as meal plans to ensure your efforts are as successful as possible.

Acknowledgments

I would like to express my gratitude to the many people who saw me through this book. Thank you to my parents, for always believing in me and encouraging me to make my dreams a reality. From the very first day when this book was simply an idea, my family's excitement and continuous support has made this journey a memorable one. Thank you to my amazing husband, Will Thomsen, who has loved and supported me from day one when I first began experimenting in the kitchen and sharing my recipes with the world on my blog. A big thank you to Nathalie Mornu for taking a chance on a new author and to Ann Barton, William Thomas, and the rest of the Alpha Books team for helping me bring my ideas to life. And finally, a special thanks to my registered dietitian support team and friends, Jessica Bringas and Catherine Young, who tested recipes and accepted samples with open arms. I am forever grateful for my family and friends who have given me the confidence to do what I love and accomplish the unimaginable.

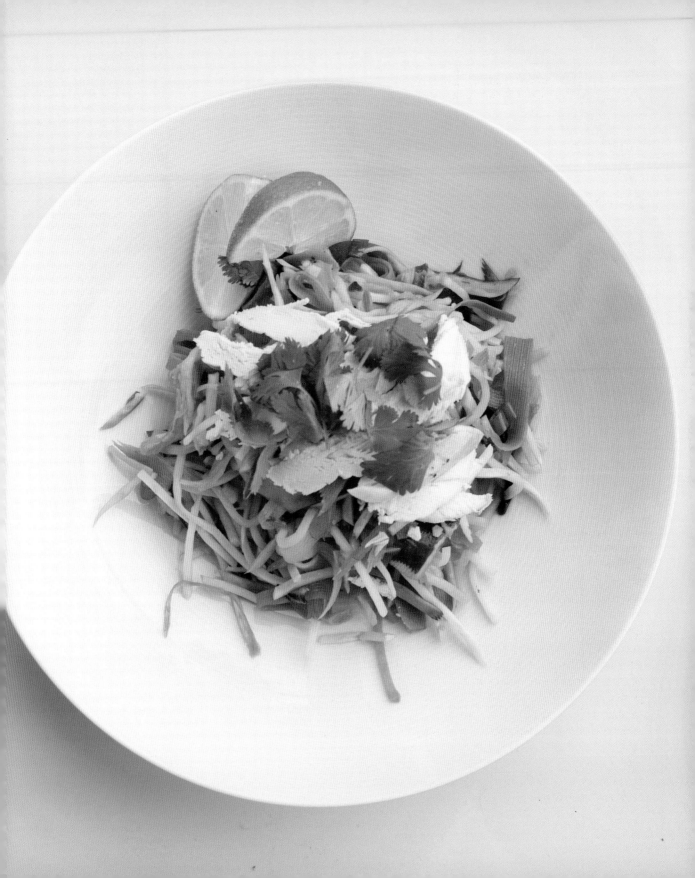

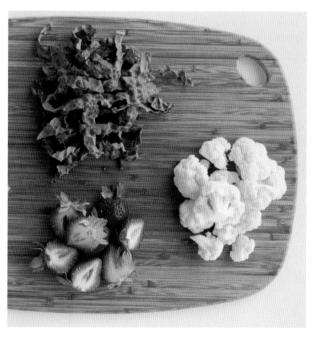
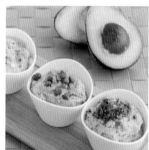
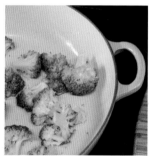

CHAPTER 1

Cooking for
Healing

What Is **Autoimmune Disease?**

Autoimmune disease can refer to a number of illnesses that are characterized by an overactive immune system that attacks the body's healthy tissues.

Abnormal Immune Response

Disorders of the immune system cause the immune system to be abnormally underactive or overactive. In cases of immune system overactivity, such as with autoimmune disorders, the body attacks and damages its own tissues.

Antibodies are response proteins that the body produces to protect us from infection. As a defense mechanism, the body's immune system naturally produces antibodies designed to fight against foreign substances that enter the body. In the case of

autoimmune disorders, however, the immune system begins producing antibodies that attack the body's own tissues. This misdirected immune system response can lead to the destruction of healthy body tissue.

Autoimmune diseases are caused by the immune system losing the ability to differentiate proteins belonging to your own body with proteins belonging to a foreign invader (like a bacteria, virus, or parasite). Which proteins or cells are selectively attacked is what differentiates one autoimmune disease from another.

Common Autoimmune Diseases

- **Alopecia areata** Immune system attacks hair follicle cells.
- **Autoimmune hepatitis** Immune system attacks the liver.
- **Celiac disease** Immune system attacks the lining of the small intestine.
- **Crohn's disease** Immune system attacks any part of the digestive tract from mouth to anus.
- **Grave's disease** Immune system attacks the thyroid, resulting in an overactive thyroid gland.
- **Hashimoto's thyroiditis** Immune system attacks the thyroid, resulting in an underactive thyroid gland.
- **Lupus** Immune system attacks cells of the skin, joints, and organs.

- **Multiple sclerosis (MS)** Immune system attacks the protective covering of nerves.
- **Pernicious anemia** Immune system attacks cells of the stomach lining; this prevents vitamin B12 from being absorbed, which is critical to producing red blood cells.
- **Psoriasis** Immune system attacks skin cells.
- **Rheumatoid arthritis** Immune system attacks the joints, particularly in the hands and feet.
- **Type 1 diabetes** Immune system attacks the pancreas, resulting in the inability to produce insulin.
- **Ulcerative colitis** Immune system attacks the lining of the large intestine (colon).

Common Symptoms

The buildup of damaged cells and tissues throughout the body in an individual with an autoimmune disease can create a variety of symptoms, such as the following:

- Allergies
- Anxiety
- Digestive problems
- Extreme fatigue
- Itchy or painful skin
- Joint and muscle pain or weakness
- Low blood pressure
- Migraines or recurrent headaches
- Numbness and tingling in extremities
- Rashes
- Reduced movement and function
- Susceptibility to infection
- Swollen glands
- Thyroid problems
- Unexplained weight changes

There are more than **80 recognized autoimmune diseases,** many of which share similar symptoms. The National Institute of Health estimates **up to 25.3 million Americans** have an autoimmune disease.

Causes and Management

Nutrient deficiencies, genetic predisposition, accidental antibody formation, and/or leaky gut are among the triggers for an autoimmune response. Leaky gut can be brought on by infection, gut dysbiosis, dietary factors, allergies or food sensitivities, medications, chronic stress, and/or inadequate sleep. Management of an autoimmune disease generally focuses on reducing immune system activity, in part by implementing dietary protocols that assist in healing a leaky gut.

What Is Leaky Gut?

Leaky gut refers to damage within your gastrointestinal tract that leads to gut permeability. What is gut permeability? Imagine a hose. When in good condition, water flows from one end of the hose to the other without leaking. If the hose becomes damaged (say we pierce the walls of the hose with a knife to create a few holes), water no longer flows seamlessly from one end to the other. Instead, due to the damage, water now leaks out of the holes. When the lining of your intestines is damaged, food no longer flows seamlessly through it. Instead, food particles leak out of the holes. However, instead of harmless water leaking out into your yard like the hose, these food particles end up in parts of your body where they don't belong. So what happens? Your immune system kicks into gear to remove these food particles so that they don't cause harm to the rest of your body. This persistent damage to the intestinal walls—commonly known as "leaky gut"—and corresponding continuous immune response is what the AIP diet is focused on repairing.

How Does **the AIP Diet** Work?

The unregulated immune system response and gut inflammation caused by autoimmune disorders can be managed with a healthy diet.

Repairing Your Gut

The autoimmune protocol (AIP) diet is a long-term health method used to address the gut inflammation that is driving an autoimmune disease. Gut inflammation causes the body to become hypersensitive to environmental triggers that an otherwise healthy person would not react to, such as certain foods.

By eliminating irritating foods that perpetuate a leaky gut and providing the body with the nourishing building blocks needed to repair the damage, this intensive healing diet allows the body to restore the balance of healthy bacteria within the gut and regulate the immune system to respond appropriately to environmental triggers, while also keeping autoimmune flare-ups at bay.

Key Nutrients

Certain vitamins and minerals support a healthy immune system and aid in decreasing inflammation throughout the body. Some of the key nutrients highlighted on the AIP diet include vitamin A, vitamin D, vitamin E, and omega-3 fatty acids.

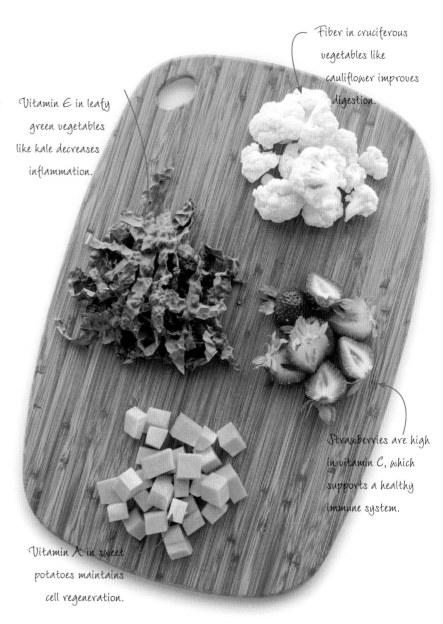

Fiber in cruciferous vegetables like cauliflower improves digestion.

Vitamin E in leafy green vegetables like kale decreases inflammation.

Strawberries are high in vitamin C, which supports a healthy immune system.

Vitamin A in sweet potatoes maintains cell regeneration.

Fueling Your Recovery

AIP-friendly foods are those that support optimal gut health. The AIP diet eliminates foods that irritate the gut, increase gut permeability, cause gut dysbiosis (an imbalance of beneficial and harmful bacteria), or activate the immune system by causing inflammation. Examples of eliminated foods include grains, legumes, dairy, eggs, nuts, seeds, and nightshade vegetables. These foods contain compounds such as lectins and alkaloids which are difficult for an inflamed, damaged gut to digest.

Additionally, the AIP diet encourages the consumption of foods that heal the gut, restore healthy gut bacteria, and regulate the immune system by decreasing inflammation. Examples of nutrient-dense foods rich in healing vitamins and minerals include non-nightshade vegetables, fruits, fish, quality meats, healthy fats, and probiotic-rich foods.

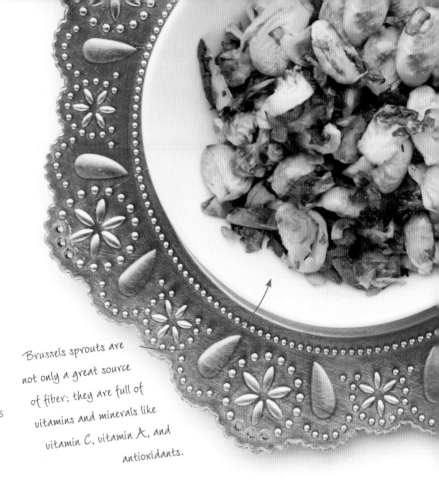

Brussels sprouts are not only a great source of fiber; they are full of vitamins and minerals like vitamin C, vitamin A, and antioxidants.

Lifestyle Factors to Support Your Diet

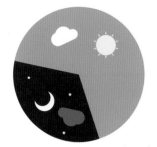

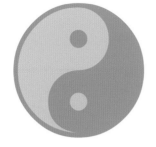

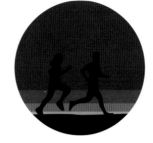

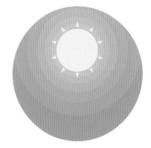

SLEEP

Giving your body time to rest is key to optimal recovery. Sleep allows your body to restore hormone levels and recharge your brain, muscles, and organs after a long day of activity and stress. Aim for at least 7 hours of sleep every night.

STRESS MANAGEMENT

Chronic stress can have negative consequences on the body. Whether it's taking a walk, spending time with friends, meditating, or keeping a thought journal, take steps to cope with stress in a healthy way.

EXERCISE

Regular physical activity can have long-term health benefits and improve your quality of life. Exercise is important to managing a healthy weight, improving mood, boosting energy levels, and promoting better sleep.

SUNLIGHT EXPOSURE

Spending time outdoors with appropriate sun exposure can increase the body's production of vitamin D. Vitamin D is important in helping the immune system function properly.

What to **Eat**

It's easy to focus on what you can't have when starting a new diet, but the AIP diet offers a robust list of delicious nutrient-dense foods to keep you satisfied.

Vegetables

- Artichoke
- Arugula
- Asparagus
- Beet
- Bok choi
- Broccoli
- Brussels sprouts
- Butternut squash
- Cabbage
- Carrot
- Cauliflower
- Celeriac/Celery root
- Celery
- Chard
- Collard greens
- Cucumber
- Fennel
- Jicama
- Kale
- Leek
- Lettuce
- Mushroom
- Onion
- Parsnip
- Pumpkin
- Radish
- Rhubarb
- Rutabaga
- Scallion
- Shallot
- Snap peas
- Spinach
- Summer squash
- Sweet potato
- Turnip
- Watercress
- Yam
- Zucchini

Fruits

- Apple
- Apricot
- Avocado
- Banana
- Blackberry
- Blueberry
- Cantaloupe
- Cherry
- Clementine
- Coconut
- Date
- Fig
- Grape
- Grapefruit
- Guava
- Honeydew
- Kiwi
- Lemon
- Lime
- Mango
- Nectarine
- Orange
- Papaya
- Peach
- Pear
- Persimmon
- Plum
- Pineapple
- Pomegranate
- Raspberry
- Strawberry
- Tangerine
- Watermelon

Meat & Poultry

- Beef
- Bison
- Chicken
- Duck
- Lamb
- Organ meat
- Pork
- Rabbit
- Turkey
- Venison

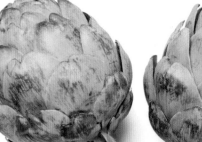

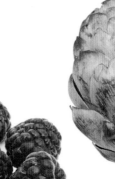

Fish & Seafood

- Catfish
- Cod
- Clams
- Crab
- Crawfish
- Flounder
- Grouper
- Halibut
- Mussels
- Oysters
- Pollock
- Salmon
- Scallops
- Sea bass
- Shrimp
- Snapper
- Sole
- Tilapia
- Tuna

Oils & Vinegars

- Apple cider vinegar
- Balsamic vinegar
- Coconut aminos
- Coconut oil
- Olive oil
- Red wine vinegar
- Sherry vinegar
- White wine vinegar

Herbs & Spices

- Basil
- Bay leaf
- Chamomile
- Chives
- Cilantro
- Cinnamon
- Cloves
- Dill
- Garlic
- Ginger
- Lavender
- Lemongrass
- Marjoram
- Mint
- Parsley
- Peppermint
- Rosemary
- Saffron
- Sage
- Sea salt
- Spearmint
- Tarragon
- Thyme
- Turmeric

Flours & Starches

- Arrowroot powder
- Coconut flour
- Tapioca starch

Condiments & Canned Goods

- Anchovies
- Baking soda
- Broths (vegetable, chicken, beef)
- Capers
- Coconut butter
- Coconut cream
- Coconut milk
- Fermented vegetables (pickles, sauerkraut, kimchi)
- Fish sauce
- Ghee*
- Lemon juice
- Lime juice
- Olives
- Purées (sweet potato, squash, pumpkin)
- Water chestnuts

Sweeteners

- Coconut sugar*
- Dried fruit*
- Honey*
- Maple syrup*
- Molasses*

Beverages

- Coconut Water
- Coffee*
- Kombucha
- Tea (black, green, herbal)*

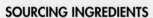

SOURCING INGREDIENTS

When shopping for ingredients, consider the following locations and resources for the best quality products.

Supermarket Find fresh produce, proteins, and pantry staples at your standard supermarkets or specialty health food store.

Farmers' Markets Get value pricing for organic produce and responsibly raised animal products at your local farmers' market.

Online Use online grocery delivery services such as U.S. Wellness Meats, Eatwild, or Amazon to purchase local or hard-to-find ingredients.

* IN MODERATION

What to **Avoid**

The AIP diet eliminates foods that irritate the gut, increase gut permeability, cause gut dysbiosis, and activate the immune system by causing inflammation.

Vegetables

- Bell pepper*
- Corn
- Eggplant*
- Hot peppers*
- Potato*
  (varieties other than sweet potatoes)
- Tomatillo*
- Tomato*

Fruits

- Goji berries*

Dairy & Eggs

- Butter
- Buttermilk
- Caesin
- Cheese
- Condensed milk
- Cottage cheese
- Cream
- Cream cheese
- Eggs
- Evaporated milk
- Frozen yogurt
- Goat cheese
- Goat milk
- Ice cream
- Kefir
- Milk
- Powdered milk
- Sheep milk
- Sour cream
- Whey protein
- Whipped cream
- Yogurt

Beans & Legumes

- Adzuki beans
- Black beans
- Black-eyed peas
- Butter beans
- Cannellini beans
- Chickpeas/ Garbanzo beans
- Fava beans/Broad beans
- Kidney beans
- Lentils
- Lima beans
- Mung beans
- Navy beans
- Peanuts
- Pinto beans
- Soybeans/ Edamame

Grains

- Amaranth
- Barley
- Buckwheat
- Bulgur
- Farro
- Kamut
- Millet
- Oats
- Quinoa
- Rice
  (all varieties)
- Rye
- Sorghum
- Spelt
- Teff
- Wheat
  (all varieties)

Nuts

- Almonds
- Brazil nuts
- Cashews
- Chestnuts
- Hazelnuts
- Macadamia nuts
- Pecans
- Pine nuts
- Pistachios
- Walnuts

What Are Nightshades?

Nightshades are a botanical family of plants that include tomatoes, potatoes, eggplants, and peppers. While most nightshades plants are inedible and actually poisonous, those that are edible contain compounds which make them a common food sensitivity and problematic for individuals with autoimmune diseases.

*INDICATES A NIGHTSHADE

Cooking with Alcohol

Some recipes in this book include wine or cognac to enhance the flavor of the finished dish. While alcohol is on the list of foods to avoid, cooking with wine or liquor over high heat allows for most of the damaging alcohol to cook off before the final product ever reaches your plate.

Seeds

- Allspice
- Anise
- Caraway
- Celery seed
- Chia seeds
- Coriander
- Cumin
- Fenugreek
- Fennel seed
- Flaxseed
- Hemp seed
- Mustard seed
- Nutmeg
- Poppy seeds
- Pumpkin seeds
- Sesame seed
- Sunflower seeds

Sweeteners

- Agave nectar
- Barley malt/Barley malt syrup
- Beet sugar
- Cane sugar
- Cane juice
- Corn syrup/Corn syrup solids
- High-fructose corn syrup
- Non-nutritive sweeteners (acesulfame potassium, aspartame, neotame, saccharin, stevia, sucralose)
- Raw sugar
- Rice syrup
- Sucanat
- Sugar alcohols (erythritol, mannitol, sorbitol, xylitol)
- Turbinado sugar

Oils & Vinegars

- Canola oil/Rapeseed oil
- Corn oil
- Cottonseed oil
- Hydrogenated or partially hydrogenated vegetable oil
- Palm kernel oil
- Peanut oil
- Safflower oil
- Soybean oil
- Sunflower oil

Other

- Alcohol
- Artificial or processed food chemicals, additives, flavorings or coloring (acrylamide, autolyzed protein, brominated vegetable oil, hydrolyzed vegetable protein, monosodium glutamate [MSG], olestra, phosphoric acid)
- Emulsifiers (carrageenan, cellulose gum, guar gum, maltodextrin, lecithin, xantham gum)
- Herbs/Spices (ashwaganda, cayenne pepper*, chili pepper flakes*, chili powder*, curry powder, paprika*)
- Soy (seitan, soy lecithin, soy sauce, tamari, tempeh, textured vegetable protein, tofu)
- Yeast

INFLAMMATORY COMPOUNDS

Many eliminated foods on the AIP diet contain the following compounds, which are difficult for an inflamed, damaged gut to digest and inhibit beneficial gut healing and restoration of healthy gut bacteria.

Lectins: These sugar-binding proteins found in nightshades protect plants from predation. The compounds are resistant to digestion, pro-inflammatory, and have the ability to increase intestinal permeability.

Alkaloids: These compounds found in nightshades can contribute to gut irritation and leaky gut.

Solanine: This compound gives potatoes their bitter taste.

Capsaicin: This compound gives peppers their heat.

Stocking Your Pantry
with Staples

Keeping your kitchen stocked with the following pantry staples will make cooking AIP-friendly recipes a breeze.

Anchovies
These small fish are great for adding flavor to dressings, sauces, and salads.

Apple cider vinegar
This vinegar is high in acetic acid which has potent antimicrobial properties.

Arrowroot powder
Extracted from the roots of the arrowroot plant, this starch can be used in baked goods or as a thickening agent.

Baking powder
Because baking powder typically contains cornstarch, make your own by substituting 1 tsp. baking powder with ½ tsp. baking soda plus ¼ tsp. cream of tartar.

Baking soda
This fine white powder acts as a leavening agent in baked goods.

Balsamic vinegar
Balsamic vinegar is made from wine vinegar blended with grape juice. The traditional sweet and sour taste makes this vinegar perfect for salad dressings, sauces, and cooked meats.

Canned seafood
Keep canned tuna, salmon, sardines, oysters, and herring on hand for a quick lunch or snack.

Capers
The edible flower bud of the caper plant is salted and pickled for use as a culinary seasoning or garnish. Capers are used in sauces, meat dishes, and salads.

Carob powder
This sweet edible pulp comes from a pod of the Mediterranean carob tree. The pulp is dried and roasted into a caffeine-free smooth powder which can be substituted for cocoa powder in nearly every recipe.

Coconut aminos
Coconut aminos is a soy-free seasoning (similar in flavor to soy sauce) that is made by fermenting coconut tree sap.

Coconut butter
Coconut butter is a thick and smooth butter made from the flesh of the coconut. It is thicker and richer than coconut oil.

Fermented Foods

Fermented foods contain naturally occurring beneficial probiotics and digestive enzymes that help boost the immune system and support a healthy gut. Whether you enjoy kombucha, pickles, or sauerkraut, read the ingredient label closely to ensure the product doesn't contain nightshades.

Coconut flour
This soft, dense flour comes from dried, ground coconut meat and can be used in baking. Because the flour is so absorbent, you only need to substitute 1 cup regular flour with about ¼ cup coconut flour.

Coconut milk and cream
Coconut milk and cream are made by combining shredded coconut with water. Coconut cream is thicker and richer in flavor than coconut milk.

Coconut oil
Coconut oil is extracted from coconut meat. This oil contains lauric acid, an easily digestible, antimicrobial fat that helps reduce inflammation. Look for unrefined virgin or pure coconut oil which has not been bleached or deodorized.

Coconut sugar
Coconut sugar is produced from the liquid sap of cut flower buds of the coconut palm tree.

Dried fruit
Keep dried fruits like raisins, dates, prunes, and apricots on hand for sweeteners in recipes or for a quick snack.

Fish sauce
Known for its savory, sweet, and umani flavors, fish sauce is extracted from fermented anchovies. Look for brands that do not contain any additional preservatives or monosodium glutamate.

Gelatin

Typically found in powder form, gelatin is derived from the collagen of animal by-products (skin, tendons, ligaments, and bones) and is commonly used in the production of jellies. It can be used as a binder in cooking or taken as a supplement to support joint health.

Ghee

Ghee, commonly referred to as clarified butter, is made by heating butter to separate and remove the milk solids which contain lactose and milk proteins. Ghee can be easily made at home or purchased commercially.

Honey

Honey can be used to sweeten dressing and desserts. Choose organic raw, unfiltered honey.

Lemon and lime juice

Purchasing presqueezed lemon and lime juices for use in dressings and sauces will save you time when it comes to food preparation.

Maple syrup

Maple syrup can be used to sweeten dressing and desserts. Try Grade B maple syrup, which has a strong maple flavor and sweet caramel undertones.

Stocks and Broths

Keep your pantry and freezer stocked with vegetable, chicken, and beef stock or broth for use in soups and stews. When purchasing store-bought broths and stocks, read the ingredients to ensure there are no artificial flavors or additives.

Molasses

Molasses can be used to sweeten sauces and baked goods. With its dark color and thick consistency, blackstrap molasses has rich flavor and superior mineral content.

Olive oil

Olive oil is a great source of healthy monounsaturated fats. Look for virgin or extra-virgin varieties.

Olives

Olives are an easy way to add flavor to a salad or meal.

Purées

Canned sweet potato, squash, and pumpkin purées can save you time in the kitchen. Use purées to thicken soups or to create a quick side dish in a pinch.

Red wine vinegar

Red wine vinegar is made from fermented and aged diluted red wine. Red wine vinegar is great for salad dressings, sauces, and pickling.

Sherry vinegar

Sherry vinegar is made from fermented sherry and adds a gourmet flavor to any vinaigrette.

Tapioca starch

Extracted from the cassava plant, this starchy white flour can be used in baked goods or as a thickening agent.

Water chestnuts

This starchy aquatic vegetable is typically found in a can and is commonly used in Asian cuisines. Its fresh taste and crunchy texture are a perfect addition to sautéed veggies or stir fries.

White wine vinegar

White wine vinegar is made from fermented and aged diluted white wine.

Coconut

You may have noticed the prevalence of coconut products that fit within the AIP diet. The versatile fruit of the coconut tree is the basis for many AIP-friendly products that can stand in for a variety of off-limits foods, including conventional flour and sugar, dairy products, and soy sauce.

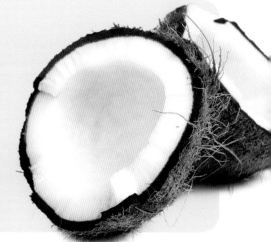

Making Good **Food Choices**

Even working within the AIP guidelines, it's easy to feel overwhelmed by the options available at your supermarket.

Reading Food Labels

Informed food choices begins with understanding food labeling. The more information you can learn about a product, the better. Look for verification symbols from the USDA and review the list of ingredients. Ingredients are listed in order of predominance, meaning that the most prevalent ingredients are listed first. Look for products with short lists of ingredients and words you recognize. If you can't pronounce an ingredient or are left with questions about the quality and sourcing of the product, avoid tossing it in your shopping cart.

Organic

According to USDA regulations, organic plants must be grown without conventional pesticides, synthetic fertilizers, sewage sludge, genetically modified ingredients, or ionizing radiation. Organic meat and poultry must come from animals that are given no antibiotics or growth hormones.

100% ORGANIC
All of the items on the ingredient list must meet the USDA organic criteria.

CERTIFIED ORGANIC
At least 95% of the items on the ingredients list must meet USDA organic criteria.

MADE WITH ORGANIC
At least 70% of the ingredients must meet the USDA organic criteria.

Natural

Refers to products that do not contain artificial ingredients or preservatives and have ingredients that are only minimally processed. Regulations for this label are more lenient than for organic labeling and natural products may still contain antibiotics and growth hormones.

Grass-Fed

Refers to animals that are raised primarily on ranges where they are allowed to graze on grass rather than the conventional grain or soy feed.

Free-Range

Refers to animals that are allowed access to the outdoors; however, the quality and size of the outdoor space, and the duration of time allotted to animals to roam outdoors, may not be regulated.

Sustainable Seafood

Refers to seafood that is either caught or farmed in a way that considers the well-being of the harvested species as well as its surrounding environment. The Monterey Bay Aquarium is a great resource for selecting the most sustainable seafood options.

Buying Organic

The Dirty Dozen list refers to conventional, non-organic fruits and vegetables that contain the highest amount of pesticide residues. Fruits and vegetables on the Clean Fifteen list contain the least amount of pesticides. When shopping for organics, prioritize items on the AIP Dirty Dozen list.

THE AIP DIRTY DOZEN	
Apple	Kale
Berries	Nectarine
Celery	Peach
Collard greens	Snap peas
Cucumber	Spinach
Grapes	Zucchini

THE AIP CLEAN FIFTEEN	
Asparagus	Kiwi
Avocado	Mango
Cabbage	Mushroom
Cantaloupe	Onion
Cauliflower	Papaya
Citrus (lemon, lime, orange, grapefruit)	Pineapple
	Sweet potato
Honeydew	Watermelon

	GOOD	BETTER	BEST
FRUITS AND VEGETABLES	Conventional fruits and vegetables	Utilizing the AIP Dirty Dozen and AIP Clean Fifteen lists	All organic, local, and seasonal produce
MEAT AND POULTRY	Antibiotic-free and hormone-free	Grass-fed and/or organic	Grass-fed, organic, and pasture-raised
SEAFOOD	Farm-raised seafood	BPA-free canned or frozen wild-caught seafood	Fresh, local, and sustainably wild-caught seafood
FATS	Conventional grain-fed ghee	Organic ghee, conventional coconut oil, conventional olive oil	Organic grass-fed lard, tallow, or ghee; organic extra-virgin coconut or olive oil
SWEETENERS	Unrefined cane sugar	Coconut sugar, conventional honey or maple syrup	Raw organic honey, organic real maple syrup

Making the Most of Your **Budget**

Eating healthy doesn't have to be expensive. Practice buying in bulk, shopping seasonally, and repurposing leftovers to make the most of your food purchases.

Buying in Bulk

The goal of buying in bulk is to reduce waste and save money. When done right, this method of shopping can yield big returns on the investment in the form of time and money.

Bulk Bins

Bulk inventory bins are becoming more and more popular at supermarkets nationwide. Look for bulk bins at your local grocery store or health food store. Bulk bins can include a variety of items such as dried spices, dried mushrooms, dried fruit, coconut flour, arrowroot powder, tapioca starch, loose teas, olive oil, vinegars, honey, and maple syrup.

Less Packaging = Money Saved

Items purchased in bulk are sold without packaging, meaning one less step for the manufacturer. This decreases the overall cost of the goods. Less packaging also means less waste and therefore a smarter environmental choice.

Price per Unit

Not all items can be purchased from open bulk bins. For items purchased frequently, look for larger packages. Scan the unit price on your favorite grocery items; you will likely notice that items purchased in a larger size or quantity typically cost less per unit than their smaller counterparts. Some supermarkets even offer discounts if purchasing items in cases. Depending on your kitchen storage space, stock up on pantry staples like broths, coconut milk, and canned fish to save time and money.

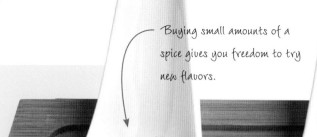

Buying small amounts of a spice gives you freedom to try new flavors.

Buy Only What You Need

Bulk bins allow you to purchase only what you need. Whether it's 1 cup or 1 teaspoon, you can avoid wasting product by scaling your purchase to the amount needed at the time of purchase.

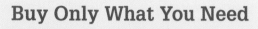

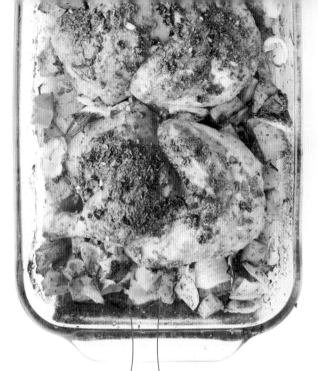

Shopping Locally and Seasonally

Local food refers to food that is grown or raised and harvested close to the consumers' homes. Because of this close proximity, the food is distributed over a much shorter distance than is common in the conventional global industrial food system. Most crops are picked at the peak of ripeness and transported directly to the store or farmstand. Therefore, local food systems are generally associated higher-quality ingredients at a lower cost. Shopping locally also allows you the opportunity to develop a personal relationship with the farmer or food processor. Ask questions about how the food is grown or raised, what sustainability measures are being executed, and details about quality control. Shopping seasonally is also important when looking for value. Purchasing foods that are in season in your area will yield the best-tasting food at the lowest cost.

Plan Ahead and Repurpose Leftovers

When batch cooking or buying in bulk, it's important to think about how these items will be used. Make time to plan how you'll use these foods in recipes and meals. For example, leftover **Greek-Style Roast Chicken** can be repurposed for making Avocado Chicken Salad or Classic Chicken and Cauliflower Soup.

Swap out sweet potatoes for summer squash, depending on the season.

Freeze individual servings of leftover chicken for quick additions to soups and salads.

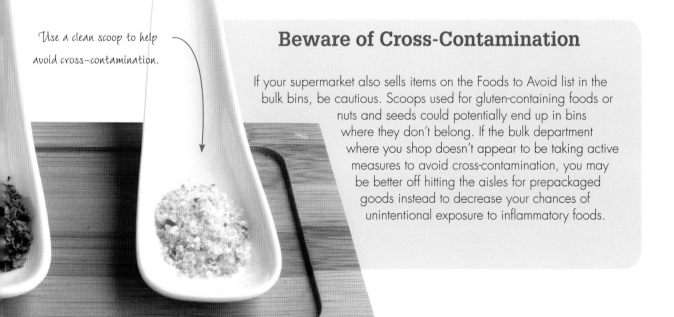

Use a clean scoop to help avoid cross-contamination.

Beware of Cross-Contamination

If your supermarket also sells items on the Foods to Avoid list in the bulk bins, be cautious. Scoops used for gluten-containing foods or nuts and seeds could potentially end up in bins where they don't belong. If the bulk department where you shop doesn't appear to be taking active measures to avoid cross-contamination, you may be better off hitting the aisles for prepackaged goods instead to decrease your chances of unintentional exposure to inflammatory foods.

Saving Time in the Kitchen

Following an AIP diet doesn't have to mean cooking every day. With planning and preparation, you can make the most of your time and ingredients.

Batch Cooking

Batch cooking refers to preparing meals and snacks ahead of time to be eaten in the future. For example, this could mean cooking on one day most or all of your meals and snacks to be eaten for the entire week ahead. By spending a few hours in your kitchen during one day out of the week, you can save yourself the headache of deciding what to make for dinner and the time of cooking everything from scratch during the week. Focus on completing the hard parts of food preparation early on to set yourself up for success when life gets busy. Batch cooking saves you time and allows you to enjoy time with loved ones, take interest in new hobbies, exercise, meditate, or decompress guilt-free, knowing that you have fueled your body optimally.

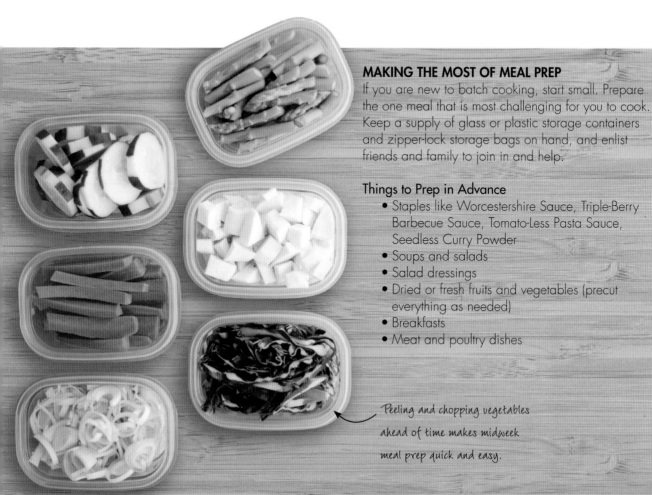

MAKING THE MOST OF MEAL PREP
If you are new to batch cooking, start small. Prepare the one meal that is most challenging for you to cook. Keep a supply of glass or plastic storage containers and zipper-lock storage bags on hand, and enlist friends and family to join in and help.

Things to Prep in Advance
- Staples like Worcestershire Sauce, Triple-Berry Barbecue Sauce, Tomato-Less Pasta Sauce, Seedless Curry Powder
- Soups and salads
- Salad dressings
- Dried or fresh fruits and vegetables (precut everything as needed)
- Breakfasts
- Meat and poultry dishes

Peeling and chopping vegetables ahead of time makes midweek meal prep quick and easy.

Meal Planning

Treat your meal plan like you would any other appointment or meeting in your life. You wouldn't blow off a meeting with your boss, so why blow off a date with your dinner plans? Plan what you are going to eat for the week and stick to it. Use the Weekly Meal Plans and Shopping Lists to help get you started. Create your own meal plan by using the tips below.

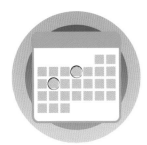

Look at your schedule.
Based on your current life commitments, determine the days and time you can commit to cooking. If you're going to be home late, plan a slow cooker meal so that the cooking can be done when you walk through the door. Knowing your schedule for the week ahead leaves little room for surprises and excuses.

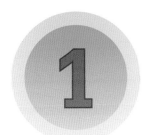

Choose ONE item for breakfast.
Buy enough ingredients for all seven days of the week and batch cook as needed on the weekend. Whether you make individual servings of Crisp Ham Cups or a batch of Apple Cinnamon Hearts Cereal, make enough to cover every morning of your week.

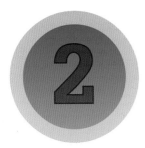

Choose TWO items to make for lunches.
Select two soup or salad recipes to use for lunches throughout the week. Make sure you have plenty of glass or plastic to-go containers and zipper-lock bags available for packing things like dressings and salad toppings.

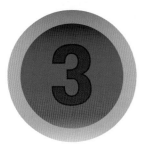

Choose THREE dinner meal ideas for dinner.
Select 3 of your favorite dinner recipes to make for dinner throughout the week. Refer to the section on Batch Cooking to help guide you in preparing ahead of time and minimize time spent in the kitchen during a busy week.

Smart Shopping

Know what you need.
Keep a running list on your refrigerator to track when your pantry staples are running low. Take this list with you on your next trip to the supermarket to ensure you never run out of the ingredients you need.

Make a detailed grocery list.
Include all of the items you will need for the week and their corresponding quantities. Take an inventory of your current freezer, refrigerator, and pantry and cross off items you already have. Add a few fresh fruits and vegetables to the list for easy grab-and-go snacks.

Go shopping.
Don't go shopping hungry. Stick to your list and don't forget any coupons and reusable grocery bags to help you save money.

Practice and have fun!
Meal planning should be fun. This is your opportunity to embrace your new AIP lifestyle, try new foods, and build your own healthy meal catalog to refer back to in the future. Ask your family members to take an active part in suggesting meals for the week.

Kitchen **Tools & Equipment**

Most of what you need to cook for an AIP diet is likely already in your kitchen. Here are some specific tools that are used throughout the book.

Special Tools

Blender A high-speed blender with a strong motor is a great investment when cooking for an AIP lifestyle. Invest in brands like Vitamix, BlendTec, and Breville and look for a model with a tamper accessory that allows you to push contents toward the blade while blending.

Electric mixer Electric mixers come in all shapes and sizes. Either a stand mixer or an inexpensive hand mixer can be used for the recipes in this book.

Food processor Choose a mid-sized (11–14 cup capacity) food processor with basic slicer and shredder discs to make everything from smooth purées to perfectly shredded slaws.

Grill pan Grill pans are great for indoor grilling all year long. Choose a ridged grill pan that is heavy-duty aluminum, stainless steel, or cast iron for consistent and even cooking. The ridges hold food up and away from the fat and juices that are rendered during cooking.

Ice pop mold Plastic ice pop molds are generally sold in sets of six ice pops and are an easy way to make your favorite frozen treats.

Juicer Juicing is a great way to obtain a large amount of nutrients in a small volume. Select a juicer that is easy to clean with pieces that are dishwasher safe.

Mandolin Choose a mandolin with a variety of blades to create uniform slices and juliennes. Look for an easily adjustable blade for creating a variety of thicknesses and a basic hand guard for safety.

Meat thermometer A meat thermometer is a lifesaver for the novice cook. Select an inexpensive digital meat thermometer and keep extra batteries on hand to ensure you know when your meat is done at all times.

Mesh sieve A mesh sieve is handy for draining steamed vegetables or straining homemade bone broths and stocks.

BLENDER   ELECTRIC MIXER   FOOD PROCESSOR   GRILL OR GRILL PAN   ICE POP MOLDS   JUICE   MANDOLIN   MEAT THERMOMETER   MESH SIEVE

Mortar and pestle A mortar and pestle comes in handy for grinding up spices quickly and easily. However, an electric spice grinder is preferred for tougher-to-handle spices.

Muffin tin While baked goods like muffins don't appear frequently on the AIP diet, a muffin tin is great for making individual-portioned entrées such as a mini meatloaves.

Oven-proof skillet A skillet has sloped slides that are larger than a traditional frying pan. An oven-proof skillet with a tight-fitting lid is most versatile.

Slow cooker A slow cooker is an indispensable appliance for anyone with a busy lifestyle. Choose a size that is compatible with your household; a 3.5–4 quart (3.5–4l) size typically feeds a family of four, while a 5–6 quart (5–6l) size is better for larger households. Programmable slow cookers that automatically switch to warm after the cooking time is complete are crucial for anyone with an unpredictable schedule.

Spiralizer A spiralizer is an inexpensive and fun kitchen tool to have on hand to make fresh veggie noodles. Look for a spiralizer with a variety of blades to make noodles of all shapes and sizes.

Stock pot or Dutch oven A large stock pot is key for making batches of soups and stews. Even better, the versatility of a Dutch oven with a tight-fitting lid allows it to be used on the stovetop and be transferred to the oven with ease.

Waffle iron An waffle iron is great for making breakfast on special occasions. Save space in the kitchen by opting for a smaller, inexpensive one for easy storage; you can always cook in batches when company visits.

Wooden skewers Use wooden skewers for kabobs and grilling. Thread your favorite meat and veggies onto moist kabobs and toss on the grill for a quick dinner.

| MORTAR & PESTLE | MUFFIN TIN | OVEN-PROOF SKILLET | SLOW COOKER | SPIRALIZER | STOCK POT OR DUTCH OVEN | WAFFLE IRON | WOODEN SKEWERS |

Other Useful Tools and Appliances

Baking pans
Baking sheets
Baster
Basting brush
Can opener
Chef's knife
Colander
Cutting boards
Dehydrator
Kitchen scissors

Ladle
Mason jars
Measuring cups (dry and liquid)
Measuring spoons
Meat tenderizer
Mixing bowls (small, medium, and large)
Peeler
Plastic squeeze bottles
Salad spinner

Saucepans
Sealable containers
Slotted spoon
Spatula
Tongs
Whisk
Wooden spoons
Zester

Ensuring Success

Adapting the AIP diet takes time. Understanding foods to avoid and adjusting to new ways of cooking can seem daunting at first. Keep these tips in mind to ensure your transition to an AIP-friendly llifestyle is as successful as possible.

Top 5 Ways to Avoid Temptation

1 Clean Out Your Pantry
Recruit your entire household to support you in your new AIP-friendly lifestyle. Remove all items from your freezer, refrigerator, and pantry that are on the **What to Avoid** food list. Non-AIP foods brought into the house by family and friends only create temptations. Keep your kitchen stocked with foods on the **What to Eat** list and leave all foods on the **What to Avoid** list on the supermarket shelves.

2 Love Your Leftovers
Temptation can strike at any time. Maybe you have a late night at the office, are unable to spend time on the weekend batch cooking due to busy family schedules, or you come home from vacation to an empty fridge. Whatever the situation is, leftovers can come in handy when managing a busy lifestyle. You can never have too many extra meals for unexpected situations. Make extra today and you will thank yourself tomorrow...or three months from now.

3 Create New Habits
If you previously ordered pizza on weekend nights or Chinese takeout every Wednesday, it's time to form new habits to avoid feeling deprived. Following an AIP diet is easier if you cook at home since you will have control over each and every ingredient within the meal. Find joy in batch cooking on the weekends and start new traditions like Soup Sundays, Slow Cooker Saturdays, or Fish Fridays.

4 Find AIP-friendly Substitutions
When sweet or salty cravings strike, be prepared. Avoid reaching for non-AIP approved foods when temptation surfaces by stocking your kitchen with ready-to-eat snacks and treats.

5 Cook for Your Family and Friends
Embrace the curiosity of your loved ones. Educate them on your new style of eating and surprise them with a delicious AIP-friendly dinner party.

Expand Your Palate

While some familiar ingredients may be off limits, grocery stores offer more variety than ever. Take advantage of new, unfamiliar ingredients and don't be afraid of something new—you never know what foods might become your new favorites! The following are some of the less-familiar fruits and vegetables you can expect to try throughout this cookbook.

- Butternut squash
- Chayote squash
- Fennel
- Ginger
- Kale
- Leeks
- Parsnips
- Pomegranate
- Portobello mushrooms
- Rutabaga
- Spaghetti squash

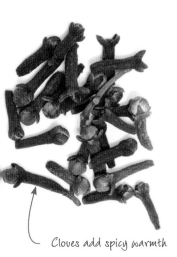

Cloves add spicy warmth to both sweet and savory dishes.

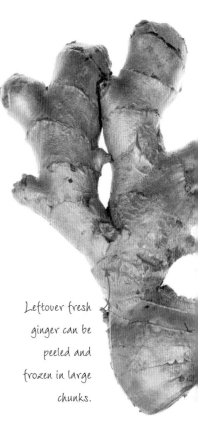

Leftover fresh ginger can be peeled and frozen in large chunks.

The Importance of Herbs and Spices

Don't just rely on salt to flavor your food. Spices and herbs add flavor, warmth, and depth to your basic ingredients and can affect the whole flavor profile of a dish. Use turmeric or ginger for an Asian-inspired cuisine. Rely on oregano and basil for an Italian twist, or garlic and cilantro for Mexican flavors.

Words of Encouragement

Start slow. Adopting an AIP lifestyle doesn't happen overnight and it's easy to become overwhelmed. Start slow and take small steps. Understanding and implementing the AIP diet is a learning process.

Embrace mistakes. Forming new eating habits can be challenging. Mistakes are inevitable. Strive for progress, not perfection.

Seek support. Nothing is more powerful than a network of support. Encourage your friends and family to try new recipes with you. Join community groups and online forums to meet individuals experiencing the same struggles.

Practice with patience. The more AIP-friendly meals you are familiar with, the easier eating and cooking for your unique condition will become. Continued practice in the kitchen will make your new eating habits become second nature.

Be prepared. You can't always predict your next meal. Whether you keep a few frozen AIP-friendly meals in the office freezer or pack dried fruit in the glove box of your car for an emergency snack, it's always better to be overly prepared.

Staple Recipes

Avoid added sugars and unwanted spices by **making your own pantry staples** from scratch.

There are many basic pantry staples we rely on to cook delicious meals. However, some of these items contain ingredients that are not AIP-friendly, such as sugar, artificial flavorings, and spices derived from seeds.

Many recipes throughout this book rely on the following staple recipes for key ingredients, which appear in boldface type on the ingredients list.

- Bone Broth
- Basic Avocado "Mayo"
- Worcestershire Sauce
- Triple-Berry Barbecue Sauce
- Tomato-Less Pasta Sauce
- Seed-Free Curry Powder

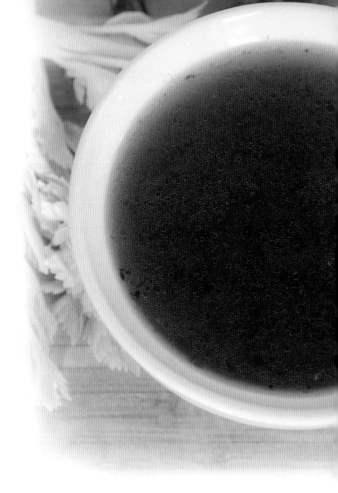

Stock Up on Staples

Save the bones from chicken, pork, and beef meals and keep a continuous collection in a zipper-lock plastic bag in the freezer until you have enough bones to make a batch of **Bone Broth**. Freeze broth in small batches or in an ice cube tray so you have easy access to the necessary portion sizes when needed.

Make several batches of **Seed-Free Curry Powder** and store it in an airtight jar in the pantry.

Freeze **Basic Avocado "Mayo"** in small batches using an ice cube tray. Thaw in the fridge overnight when ready to use.

Prepare a few batches of **Triple-Berry Barbecue Sauce** and **Tomato-Less Pasta Sauce** and freeze them in small containers for use as needed.

Worcestershire Sauce can be made ahead and kept in the refrigerator for up to one month.

This **mineral-rich savory broth** can be used as a base for soups or stews, or consumed as a beverage for a quick nutritious boost.

Bone Broth

 YIELD: **6 CUPS**   SERVING SIZE: **1 CUP**   PREP TIME: **5 MINUTES**   COOK TIME: **24 HOURS**

INGREDIENTS

- 2 roasted chicken carcasses (about 1 ½ lbs. [680g] of bones)
- 2 stalks celery, chopped into large chunks
- 2 carrots, unpeeled and chopped into large chunks
- 1 medium yellow onion, unpeeled and quartered
- 1 head garlic, sliced, unpeeled and halved lengthwise
- 1 bay leaf
- 5–10 sprigs fresh thyme
- 5–10 sprigs fresh parsley
- 2 TB. apple cider vinegar
- 6 cups water
- Salt

METHOD

1 Place bones, celery, and carrots in a slow cooker. Add onion, garlic, bay leaf, thyme, and parsley.

3 Add apple cider vinegar and enough water to cover all of the bones and vegetables. Cook on low for 24 hours.

4 Using a slotted spoon, remove and discard the vegetables and bones.

5 Using a fine mesh sieve, strain the broth into a large container or several small containers. Cover and refrigerate overnight or until chilled.

6 Scrape fat from the top of the broth and discard. Taste and season with salt as needed.

Storage: After removing the fat layer from the broth, store in the refrigerator for up to 1 week or freeze for up to 6 months.

You can use any mix of beef, pork, or chicken bones for making bone broth. Adding meaty bones such as short ribs or ham bones will add extra flavor to your broth.

SPECIAL TOOLS

 SLOW COOKER

 MESH SIEVE

NUTRITION

Calories 86
Total Fat 3g
Saturated Fat 1g
Unsaturated Fat 2g
Cholesterol 7mg
Sodium 45mg
Carbohydrate 0g
Dietary Fiber 0g
Sugar 0g
Protein 6g

In this versatile recipe, tart apple cider vinegar and lemon juice accompany the **creamy texture of the avocado** to create the perfect mayonnaise substitute.

Basic **Avocado "Mayo"**

 YIELD: **1 CUP**   SERVING SIZE: **2 TB.**   PREP TIME: **10 MINUTES**   COOK TIME: **NONE**

INGREDIENTS

1 medium avocado

2 TB. apple cider vinegar

2 TB. olive oil

2¼ tsp. lemon juice

½ tsp. salt

SPECIAL TOOLS

 FOOD PROCESSOR

METHOD

1 Cut avocado in half and discard the pit. Scoop avocado flesh from skin and place in a food processor.

2 Add apple cider vinegar, olive oil, lemon juice, and salt. Process for 30 seconds or until smooth.

Storage: Store in an airtight container for up to 3 days or freeze in an ice cube tray for single serving use for up to 3 months.

Serving suggestion: Dip Rosemary Sweet Potato Chips into Garlic Herb Mayo, drizzle Wasabi Avocado Mayo over Honey Ginger Glazed Salmon or serve Sweet Potato Chip Fish Sticks with a side of Tartar Sauce Mayo.

Variations: For **Garlic Herb Avocado Mayo,** add 2 garlic cloves, 2 TB. fresh parsley, 2 TB. fresh rosemary, and 2 TB. fresh thyme.

For **Wasabi Avocado Mayo,** add 2 tsp. wasabi powder and 1½ tsp. coconut aminos.

For **Tartar Sauce Mayo,** substitute apple cider vinegar for white wine vinegar and add ½ cup chopped dill pickles, 2 TB. capers, and ¼ tsp. fresh horseradish.

Use this AIP-friendly mayo for any recipe that calls for regular mayo to avoid processed oils, eggs, and dairy.

NUTRITION

Calories 76

Total Fat 8g

Saturated Fat 1g

Unsaturated Fat 6g

Cholesterol 0mg

Sodium 147mg

Carbohydrate 3g

Dietary Fiber 2g

Sugar 0g

Protein 1g

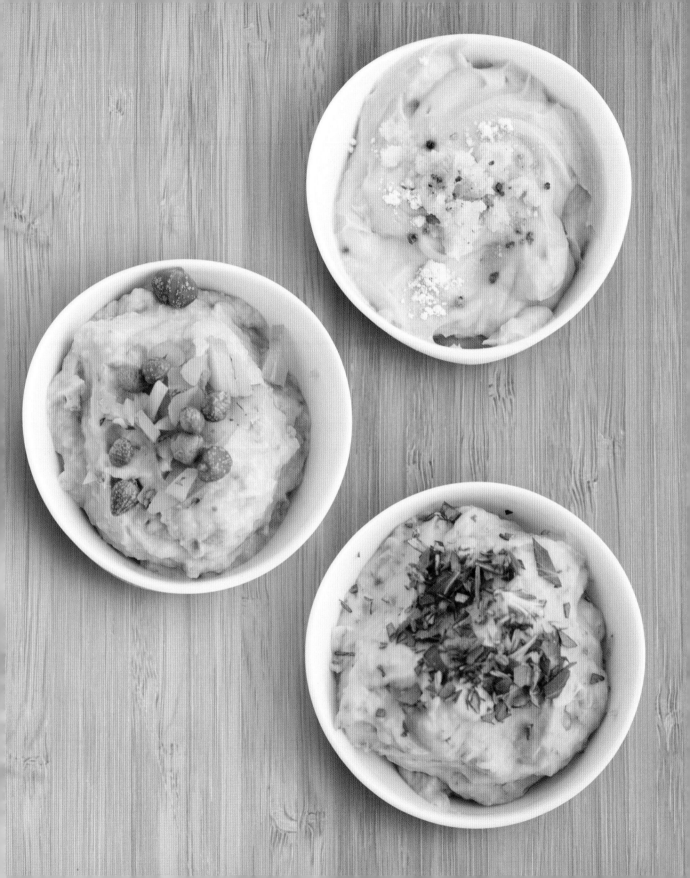

Like the store-bought version, this quick and easy sauce is **bursting with bold, sweet, sour, and salty flavors**, but it uses only AIP-friendly ingredients.

Worcestershire Sauce

 YIELD: **½ CUP**   SERVING SIZE: **1 TSP.**   PREP TIME: **3 MINUTES**   COOK TIME: **NONE**

INGREDIENTS

½ cup apple cider vinegar

2 TB. fish sauce

1 TB. honey

1 TB. molasses

1 TB. lime juice

¼ tsp. ground cloves

¼ tsp. garlic powder

½ tsp. onion powder

METHOD

1 In a blender or food processor, combine apple cider vinegar, fish sauce, honey, molasses, lime juice, ground cloves, garlic powder, and onion powder.

2 Process for 30 seconds or until smooth and combined.

Storage: Store in an airtight container in the refrigerator for up to 1 month.

Fish sauce is an umami-rich flavoring agent extracted from salted and fermented anchovies. Be sure to select a brand without added sugar.

SPECIAL TOOLS

 BLENDER

NUTRITION

Calories 7	Saturated Fat 0g	Cholesterol 0g	Carbohydrate 2g	Sugar 1g
Total Fat 0g	Unsaturated Fat 0g	Sodium 125g	Dietary Fiber 0g	Protein 0g

This **smoky and sweet barbecue sauce** is completely nightshade free. Bacon fat and Worcestershire Sauce add depth and tangy flavor.

Triple-Berry **Barbecue Sauce**

 YIELD: **2 CUPS**   SERVING SIZE: **¼ CUP**   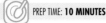 PREP TIME: **10 MINUTES**   COOK TIME: **15 MINUTES**

INGREDIENTS

1 TB. bacon fat

2 cups yellow onion, chopped (1 large onion)

1 cup carrots, peeled and chopped (2 large carrots)

3 cloves garlic, minced

⅓ cup strawberries, chopped

⅓ cup cherries, pitted

⅓ cup blueberries

¼ cup maple syrup

3 TB. **Worcestershire Sauce**

1 TB. apple cider vinegar

2 TB. coconut aminos

2 TB. molasses

½ cup beef broth

½ tsp. smoked sea salt

SPECIAL TOOLS

 BLENDER

METHOD

1 In a medium saucepan, combine bacon fat, onion, carrots, and garlic. Cook for 5 minutes over medium-high heat or until vegetables begin to soften.

2 Add strawberries, cherries, blueberries, maple syrup, Worcestershire Sauce, apple cider vinegar, coconut aminos, molasses, beef broth, and smoked sea salt.

3 Stir to combine and bring contents to a boil. Reduce heat and simmer for 10 minutes.

4 Transfer contents to a high-speed blender and blend until smooth.

Storage: Store sauce in an airtight jar or squeeze bottle for up to 2 weeks.

Serving suggestion: Use with Triple-Berry Barbecue Ribs or New Orleans Barbecue Shrimp, or mix into Orange Pulled Pork Carnitas for an easy barbecue pulled pork.

NUTRITION

Calories 109

Total Fat 2g

Saturated Fat 1g

Unsaturated Fat 1g

Cholesterol 2mg

Sodium 114mg

Carbohydrate 23g

Dietary Fiber 2g

Sugar 16g

Protein 1g

With red beets, creamy sweet potatoes, and savory onion and garlic, this **tomato-free sauce has all of the flavors you love,** without the nightshades.

Tomato-Less **Pasta Sauce**

 YIELD: **2 CUPS**   SERVING SIZE: **½ CUP** 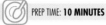 PREP TIME: **10 MINUTES**   COOK TIME: **20 MINUTES**

INGREDIENTS

2 TB. olive oil

2 cups yellow onion, chopped (1 large onion)

4 garlic cloves, minced

1 cup carrot, chopped

½ cup celery, chopped

1 TB. beet, peeled and finely chopped

1 TB. balsamic vinegar

4 tsp. lemon juice

2 TB. sweet potato purée

1 tsp. dried basil

1 tsp. dried thyme

1 tsp. dried oregano

½ tsp. salt

2 cups vegetable broth

SPECIAL TOOLS

 BLENDER

METHOD

1 Heat a large saucepan over medium-high heat. Add oil, onion, garlic, carrot, celery, and beet. Sauté for 5 minutes or until the vegetables begin to soften.

2 Add balsamic vinegar, lemon juice, sweet potato purée, ½ tsp. basil, ½ tsp. thyme, ½ tsp. oregano, salt, and vegetable broth.

3 Bring sauce to a boil, reduce heat, and cover. Simmer for 10 minutes.

4 Remove pan from heat. In a high-speed blender, blend sauce until smooth.

5 Return sauce to pan and add remaining ½ tsp. basil, ½ tsp. thyme, and ½ tsp. oregano.

Storage: Store sauce in an airtight container in the refrigerator for 1 week or freeze for up to 3 months.

Serving Suggestion: Serve sauce over Herbed Baked Spaghetti Squash with Pork and Fennel Meatballs for a quick dinner, or add to your favorite soup or stew recipe for a burst of umami flavor.

NUTRITION

Calories 132

Total Fat **7g**

Saturated Fat **1g**

Unsaturated Fat **6g**

Cholesterol **0mg**

Sodium **619mg**

Carbohydrate **16g**

Dietary Fiber **3g**

Sugar **7g**

Protein **2g**

Like traditional curry powders, this **curry powder alternative** is savory and robust. It will add a **bold, spicy flavor** to almost any dish.

Seed-Free **Curry Powder**

 YIELD: **2½ TB.**   SERVING SIZE: **1½ TSP.**   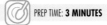 PREP TIME: **3 MINUTES**   COOK TIME: **NONE**

INGREDIENTS

1½ tsp. onion powder

1½ tsp. garlic powder

1½ tsp. dried turmeric

1 tsp. dried cilantro

1 tsp. dried basil

½ tsp. dried dill weed

½ tsp. ground cinnamon

½ tsp. ground ginger

¼ tsp. ground cloves

METHOD

1 In a mortar and pestle or spice grinder, combine onion powder, garlic powder, turmeric, cilantro, basil, dill weed, cinnamon, ginger, and cloves

2 Grind to a fine powder. Once you have reached the desired consistency, transfer to an airtight container.

Storage: Store in an airtight container away from heat and light for up to 6 months.

SPECIAL TOOLS

 MORTAR AND PESTLE

NUTRITION

Calories 10	Saturated Fat 0g	Cholesterol 0mg	Carbohydrate 2g	Sugar 1g
Total Fat 0g	Unsaturated Fat 0g	Sodium 2mg	Dietary Fiber 1g	Protein 0g

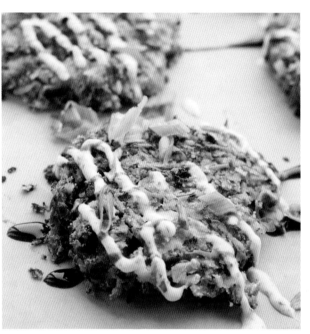

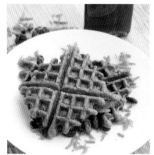

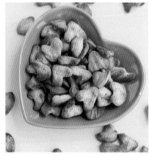

CHAPTER 2

Breakfast

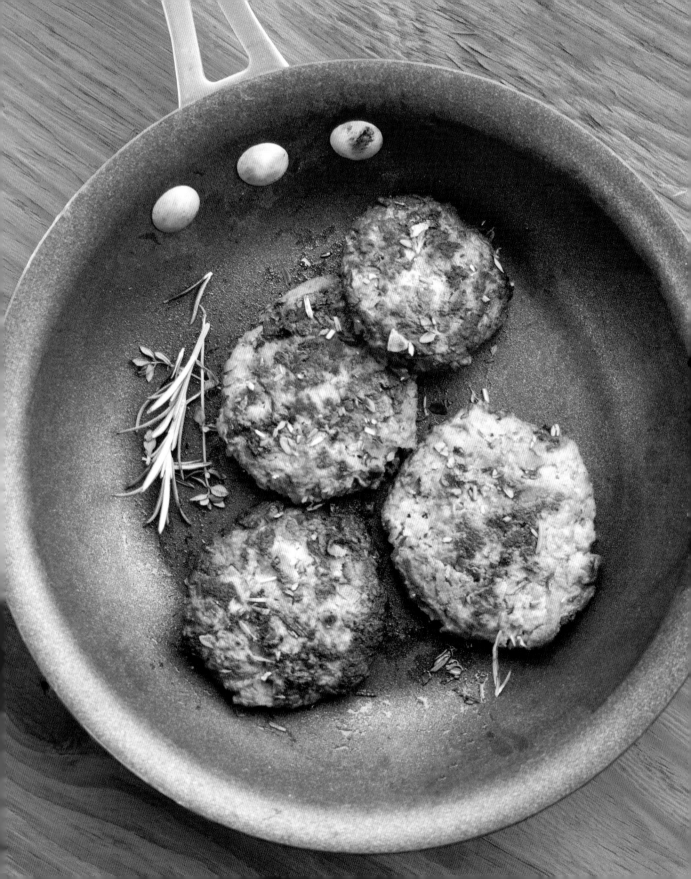

Shredded apples and a **hint of maple syrup** give these herbed pork sausage patties a sweet breakfast flavor.

Rosemary and Thyme
Breakfast Sausage Patties

 YIELD: **12 PATTIES**   SERVING SIZE: **1 PATTY**   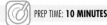 PREP TIME: **10 MINUTES**   COOK TIME: **10 MINUTES**

INGREDIENTS

1 lb. (450g) ground pork

1 TB. maple syrup

1 tsp. sea salt

1 tsp. fresh rosemary, chopped

1 tsp. fresh thyme, chopped

1 TB. fresh sage, chopped

2 cups Granny Smith apple, peeled and grated (1 large apple)

1 cup yellow onion, chopped

1 clove garlic, minced

1 TB. olive oil

METHOD

1 In a large mixing bowl, combine pork, maple syrup, sea salt, rosemary, thyme, sage, apple, onion, and garlic. With clean hands, mix ingredients until well combined.

2 Shape ½-cup portions of meat mixture into firm patties.

3 Place a skillet over medium-high heat. Add olive oil to pan and swirl to coat.

4 Add patties to skillet in batches, being careful not to crowd the pan. Cover and fry each batch for 3 minutes. Flip and cook on other side for another 3 minutes.

Storage: Sausage patties can be refrigerated for up to 1 week or frozen for up to 3 months.

Serving Suggestion: Serve sausage patties with Root Vegetable Breakfast Hash.

NUTRITION

Calories 114	Saturated Fat 3g	Cholesterol 27mg	Carbohydrate 4g	Sugar 3g
Total Fat 8g	Unsaturated Fat 5g	Sodium 218mg	Dietary Fiber 1g	Protein 6g

This **sweet breakfast** staple features cauliflower in place of oats. With flavors of apple, cinnamon, and coconut, it is **perfect for any chilly morning**.

Apple Cinnamon
No-Oat Oatmeal

 YIELD: **1 CUP**   SERVING SIZE: **½ CUP**   PREP TIME: **5 MINUTES**   COOK TIME: **25 MINUTES**

INGREDIENTS

1 cup cauliflower florets

1 cup light coconut milk

½ cup unsweetened applesauce

¼ cup unsweetened shredded coconut

2 TB. maple syrup

½ tsp. vanilla extract

½ tsp. cinnamon

⅛ tsp. ground cloves

Dash salt

SPECIAL TOOLS

 FOOD PROCESSOR

METHOD

1 Place cauliflower in a food processor. Pulse until it is finely chopped and has a rice-like consistency.

2 Transfer cauliflower rice to a small saucepan. Add coconut milk, applesauce, shredded coconut, maple syrup, vanilla extract, cinnamon, cloves, and salt. Stir to combine.

3 Bring contents to a boil over medium-high heat. Reduce heat to medium-low, cover, and simmer for 20 minutes or until mixture has thickened.

4 Return cauliflower mixture to a clean food processor and process for 30 seconds to create a smoother consistency.

5 Allow porridge to cool for 5 minutes before serving.

Storage: Store in an airtight container and refrigerate for up to 1 week.

Serving Suggestion: Served at room temperature with chopped fresh apples or raisins.

Save time by cooking in batches. Process the entire head of cauliflower and save ½-cup servings of cauliflower rice in the refrigerator to create this tasty breakfast with ease throughout the week.

NUTRITION

Calories 202	Saturated Fat 3g	Cholesterol 0mg	Carbohydrate 30g	Sugar 24g
Total Fat 9g	Unsaturated Fat 0g	Sodium 88mg	Dietary Fiber 4g	Protein 1g

Sweet, tart, and silky smooth, this dairy-free "yogurt" marries nutrient-rich avocados with the delicious flavors of **key lime pie**.

Key Lime Avocado **No'gurt**

 YIELD: **2 CUPS**   SERVING SIZE: **⅔ CUP**   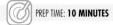 PREP TIME: **10 MINUTES**   COOK TIME: **1 HOUR**

INGREDIENTS

2 cups avocado (2 medium avocados)

7 TB. maple syrup

2 TB. lime juice

1 TB. lime zest (1 small lime)

SPECIAL TOOLS

 FOOD PROCESSOR

METHOD

1 Cut avocado in half and discard the pit. Scoop avocado flesh from the skin and place in a food processor fitted with a chopping blade.

2 Add maple syrup, lime juice, and lime zest to the food processor. Process for 30 seconds or until smooth.

3 Transfer to a small bowl and refrigerate for 1 hour before serving.

Storage: Store in an airtight container and refrigerate for up to 3 days.

Serving Suggestion: Top No'gurt with unsweetened coconut flakes or fresh berries.

Variation: For Zesty Lemon Avocado No'gurt, substitute lemon juice for lime juice and add lemon zest instead of lime zest.

In addition to their gorgeous green color, avocados are extremely nutrient-dense, meaning they pack plenty of vitamins, minerals, and phytonutrients into each and every calorie.

NUTRITION

Calories 286	Saturated Fat 2g	Cholesterol 0mg	Carbohydrate 42g	Sugar 33g
Total Fat 15g	Unsaturated Fat 12g	Sodium 10mg	Dietary Fiber 7g	Protein 2g

This **sweet and crunchy cereal** is made with all AIP-friendly ingredients, including coconut flour, unsweetened **applesauce**, and ground **cinnamon**.

Apple Cinnamon Hearts **Cereal**

 YIELD: **4 CUPS**   SERVING SIZE: **½ CUP**   PREP TIME: **20 MINUTES**   COOK TIME: **15 MINUTES**

INGREDIENTS

½ cup coconut flour

½ cup arrowroot powder

¼ cup coconut oil

1 cup unsweetened applesauce

2 tsp. vanilla extract

¼ cup maple syrup

1 tsp. ground cinnamon

SPECIAL TOOLS

 BLENDER

METHOD

1 Preheat oven to 375°F (190°C). Line a baking sheet with parchment paper.

2 In a blender, combine coconut flour, arrowroot powder, coconut oil, applesauce, vanilla, 2 tablespoons maple syrup, and cinnamon. Blend for 30 seconds or until smooth.

2 Transfer batter into a zipper-lock bag. Cut a small hole in the corner of the bag to allow batter to piped out.

3 Pipe batter into small heart shapes directly onto parchment paper, continuing until all batter is used.

4 Bake for 10 minutes. Remove pan from the oven and drizzle with additional 2 tablespoons maple syrup. Return to oven and bake for another 5 minutes.

5 Remove pan from oven and let cereal cool completely on pan.

Storage: Store at room temperature in an airtight container for up to 1 week.

Serving Suggestion: Serve with cold coconut milk or as a crunchy topping for Key Lime Avocado No'gurt.

NUTRITION

| Calories 159 | Saturated Fat 13g | Cholesterol 0mg | Carbohydrate 19g | Sugar 9g |
| Total Fat 8g | Unsaturated Fat 1g | Sodium 9mg | Dietary Fiber 3g | Protein 2g |

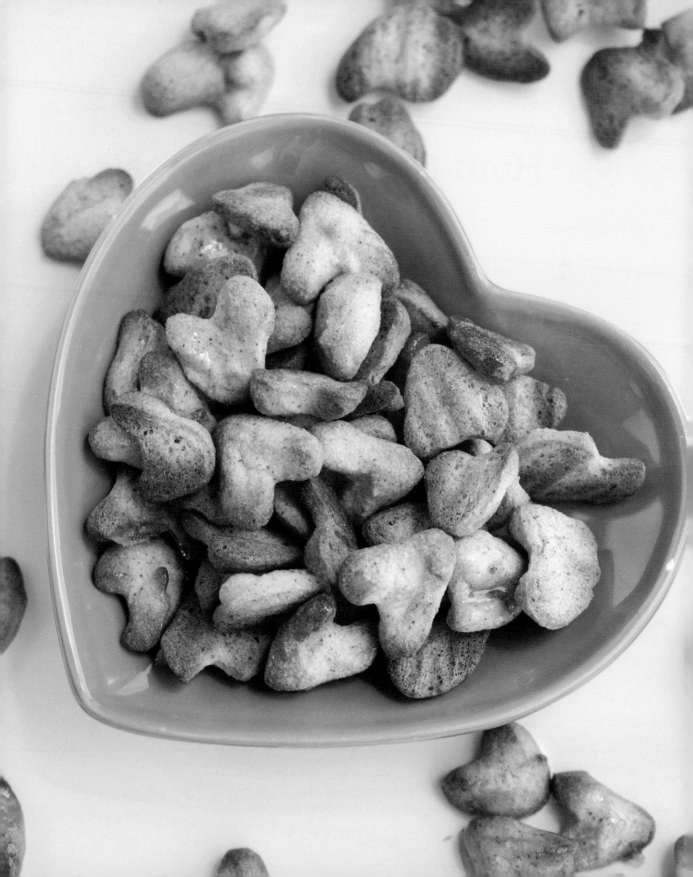

Slices of deli ham are formed into **crisp, savory cups** perfect for filling with vegetable hash for an easy **grab-and-go breakfast**.

Crisp **Ham Cups**

 YIELD: **12 HAM CUPS**   SERVING SIZE: **2 HAM CUPS**   PREP TIME: **2 MINUTES**   COOK TIME: **20 MINUTES**

INGREDIENTS

12 slices deli ham

SPECIAL TOOLS

 12-CUP MUFFIN PAN

METHOD

1 Preheat oven to 350°F (180°C).

2 Spray muffin pan with olive oil nonstick cooking spray.

3 Line each muffin cup with a slice of ham, forming the ham into a cup shape.

4 Bake for 10 minutes. Rotate pan and bake for another 10 minutes until crisp and golden brown.

Storage: These are best served crisp right out of the oven, but can be refrigerated for up to 48 hours.

Serving Suggestion: Serve filled with Root Vegetable Breakfast Hash.

NUTRITION

| Calories 82 | Saturated Fat 1g | Cholesterol 35mg | Carbohydrate 35g | Sugar 0g |
| Total Fat 1g | Unsaturated Fat 0g | Sodium 467mg | Dietary Fiber 0g | Protein 14g |

Colorful purple sweet potatoes, **sweet** carrots, **spicy** parsnips, and **savory** rutabaga make a nutrient-rich alternative to traditional **hash browns**.

Root Vegetable **Breakfast Hash**

 YIELD: **2 CUPS**   SERVING SIZE: ½ **CUP**   PREP TIME: **10 MINUTES**   COOK TIME: **15 MINUTES**

INGREDIENTS

2 TB. bacon fat

1 cup purple sweet potato, peeled and chopped

1 TB. shallot, chopped

1 cup yellow onion, chopped (½ onion)

½ cup carrots, peeled and chopped

½ cup parsnips, peeled and chopped

1 cup rutabaga, peeled and chopped

1 tsp. fresh rosemary, chopped

1 tsp. fresh thyme, chopped

½ tsp. fresh chives, chopped

⅛ tsp. sea salt

METHOD

1 In a large skillet, heat bacon fat over medium-high heat.

2 Add sweet potato, shallot, onion, carrots, parsnips, and rutabaga.

3 Cook for 10 minutes. Cover pan and continue cooking for another 5 minutes or until vegetables are fork tender.

4 Sprinkle rosemary, thyme, chives, and sea salt over vegetables and stir to combine.

Storage: Refrigerate for up to 3 days or freeze for up to 3 months.

Serving Suggestion: Spoon hash into Crisp Ham Cups for a quick and easy breakfast.

Purple sweet potato has deep purple skin and vibrant purple flesh. Its flavor is similar to that of its orange cousin, so a regular sweet potato can be substituted in this recipe if needed.

NUTRITION

Calories 162	Saturated Fat 3g	Cholesterol 6mg	Carbohydrate 24g	Sugar 5g
Total Fat 7g	Unsaturated Fat 4g	Sodium 103mg	Dietary Fiber 4g	Protein 2g

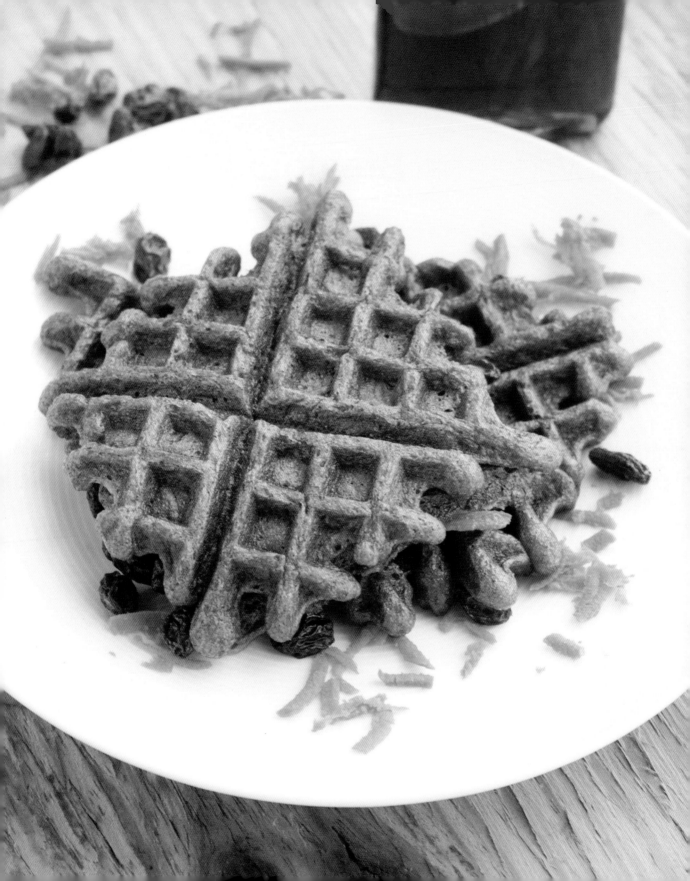

Shredded carrots and raisins bring classic carrot cake flavor to these tender waffles made with plantains, pumpkin purée, and sweet maple syrup.

Carrot Cake **Waffles**

 YIELD: **12 WAFFLES**   SERVING SIZE: **2 WAFFLES**   PREP TIME: **15 MINUTES**   COOK TIME: **2 MINUTES**

INGREDIENTS

- 3 cups plantains, peeled and chopped (ripe or green)
- ½ cup pumpkin purée
- ¼ cup coconut oil, melted
- ¼ cup maple syrup
- ½ cup light coconut milk
- 1 tsp. apple cider vinegar
- ½ cup arrowroot powder
- 2 tsp. baking soda
- 1 tsp. cream of tartar
- 1 tsp. ground cinnamon
- ½ tsp. ground ginger
- 1 cup shredded carrots
- ½ cup raisins

METHOD

1 Combine plantains, pumpkin purée, coconut oil, maple syrup, coconut milk, and apple cider vinegar in a blender. Blend until smooth.

2 Add arrowroot powder, baking soda, cream of tartar, cinnamon, and ginger to blender. Blend until smooth.

3 Transfer batter to a large bowl. Fold in shredded carrots and raisins.

4 Heat waffle iron on medium heat. Spoon a ¼-cup portion of batter into a well-greased waffle iron and cook for 2 to 3 minutes. Continue with remaining batter, greasing waffle iron between batches.

Storage: Waffles are best served immediately, but can be stored in the freezer for up to 1 month and reheated in a toaster.

Serving Suggestion: Top waffles with Coconut Whipped Cream or maple syrup.

SPECIAL TOOLS

 BLENDER

 WAFFLE MAKER

NUTRITION

Calories 319
Total Fat **11g**
Saturated Fat **16g**
Unsaturated Fat **1g**
Cholesterol **0mg**
Sodium **445mg**
Carbohydrate **56g**
Dietary Fiber **4g**
Sugar **30g**
Protein **2g**

With **toasted coconut** as a base, this **AIP-friendly breakfast cereal** is free of grains and nuts but retains the texture and flavor of traditional granola.

Sweet and Spicy **Gra'no'la**

 YIELD: **3 CUPS**   SERVING SIZE: **½ CUP**   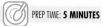 PREP TIME: **5 MINUTES**   COOK TIME: **10 MINUTES**

INGREDIENTS

1 TB. coconut oil

1 TB. coconut butter

2 cups unsweetened coconut flakes

½ tsp. cinnamon

¼ tsp. sea salt

½ tsp. coconut sugar

½ cup unsweetened banana chips, chopped

½ cup unsweetened dried mango, chopped

METHOD

1 Preheat oven to 350°F (180°C).

2 In a small saucepan over low heat, combine coconut oil and coconut butter. Stir until melted. Remove from heat and set aside.

3 In a large bowl, combine coconut flakes, coconut oil mixture, cinnamon, salt, and coconut sugar. Toss to combine until the flakes are well coated.

4 Line a baking sheet with parchment paper. Spread coconut flakes on baking sheet and bake for 5 minutes. With a spatula, stir coconut flakes and bake for another 2 to 3 minutes or until golden brown.

5 Remove coconut flakes from oven and transfer to an airtight container. Cool, uncovered, in refrigerator or freezer for 10 minutes until dry.

6 Add banana chips and dried mango to coconut flakes. Mix to combine.

Storage: Refrigerate or freeze in a covered, airtight container for up to 1 week.

Serving Suggestion: Sprinkle granola over Key Lime Avocado No'gurt or serve with chilled coconut milk.

NUTRITION

Calories 210

Total Fat 13g

Saturated Fat 10g

Unsaturated Fat 0g

Cholesterol 0mg

Sodium 116mg

Carbohydrate 15g

Dietary Fiber 3g

Sugar 10g

Protein 1g

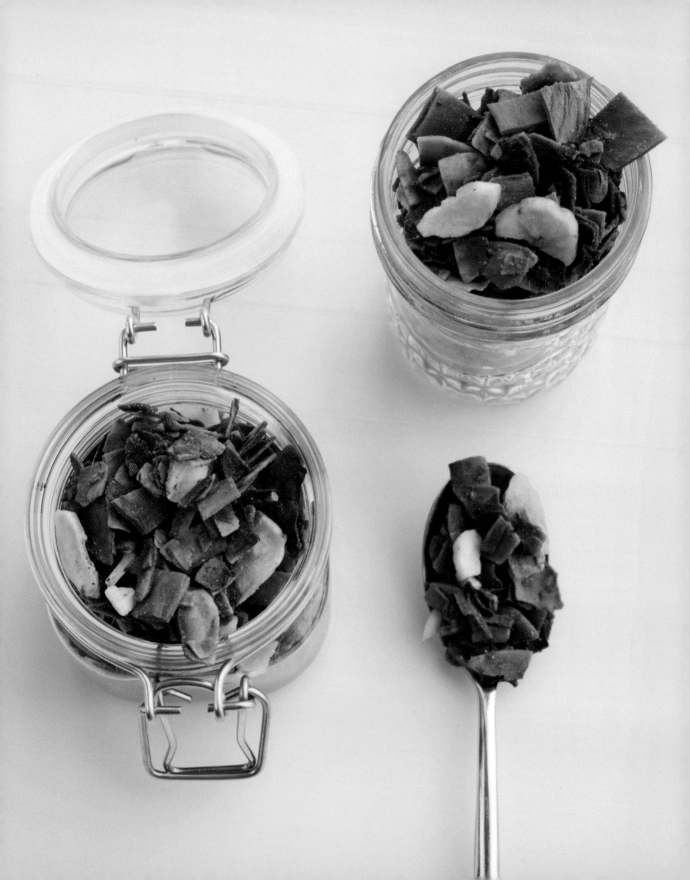

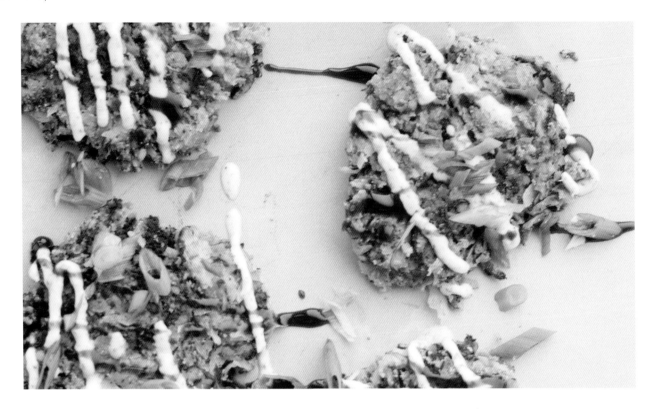

Egg Substitutes

Eggs act as binding agents in many recipes. However, on the AIP diet, eggs are on the avoid list. Try one of these egg alternatives when adapting recipes for an AIP lifestyle.

Unsweetened applesauce: Depending on the recipe, applesauce can add sweetness and moisture to a dish, like in these savory vegetable pancakes.

Plantains: The gummy texture of mashed plantains or bananas makes a great egg replacement. Use ¼ cup ripe banana or plantain in place of 1 egg. Make Carrot Cake Waffles to give this substitute a try.

Tapioca starch: When mixed with water and heated, tapioca starch develops a thick, glue-like consistency. In a small saucepan, whisk together 2½ teaspoons tapioca starch and 1 cup water. Bring contents to a boil, whisking constantly for 30 seconds. Set aside to cool until it thickens. Use 3 tablespoons in place of 1 egg.

Gelatin: Substitute gelatin for eggs to lend a chewy texture to your baked goods, such as Flourless Brownies. In place of one egg, combine 1 tablespoon gelatin with 3 tablespoons hot water and whisk until frothy.

Substitute ¼ cup applesauce for 1 egg in baked goods.

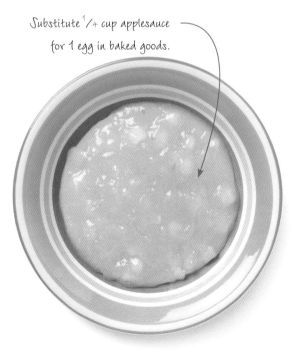

These savory Japanese **vegetable pancakes** rely on the binding properties of **coconut flour and applesauce** to form tasty, nutrient-dense fritters.

Okonomiyaki
(Savory Japanese Pancake)

 YIELD: **10 PANCAKES**   SERVING SIZE: **2 PANCAKES**   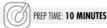 PREP TIME: **10 MINUTES**   COOK TIME: **20 MINUTES**

INGREDIENTS

3 cups cabbage (any variety), shredded

1 cup zucchini, shredded

1 cup carrots, shredded

½ cup green onions, chopped

⅓ cup coconut flour

1 tsp. arrowroot powder

1 (13.5-oz; 400ml) can light coconut milk

¼ tsp. **Seed-Free Curry Powder**

¼ tsp. sea salt

¼ tsp. garlic powder

⅓ cup unsweetened applesauce

1 TB. coconut oil

METHOD

1 In a large bowl, combine cabbage, zucchini, carrots, and green onions.

2 In a small bowl, combine coconut flour, arrowroot powder, coconut milk, Seed-Free Curry Powder, salt, garlic powder, and applesauce.

3 Pour the wet ingredients over the vegetable mixture and gently mix to combine.

4 Heat coconut oil in a large skillet over medium-high heat. Scoop ¼-cup spoonfuls of batter into hot pan.

5 Cook for 5 minutes. Carefully holding the pancakes together, flip and cook for another 5 minutes on the other side until golden brown.

Storage: Okonomiyaki is best served immediately.

Serving Suggestion: Top with Coconut Cream Ranch Dressing and garnish with additional green onions.

NUTRITION

Calories 172

Total Fat 8g

Saturated Fat 8g

Unsaturated Fat 0g

Cholesterol 0mg

Sodium 175mg

Carbohydrate 19g

Dietary Fiber 7g

Sugar 8g

Protein 4g

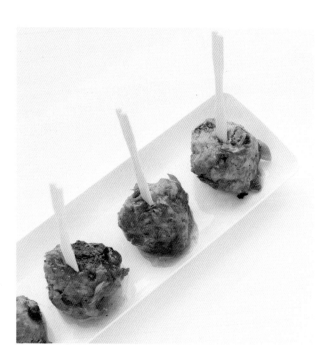
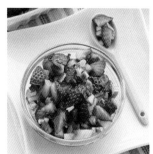
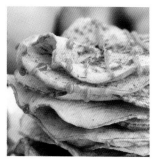

CHAPTER 3

Appetizers
& Snacks

Tangy and sweet apricot preserves pair with the **savory flavors of ginger and garlic** to create a hearty appetizer perfect for any cocktail party.

Sweet & Sour
Cocktail Meatballs

 YIELD: **32 MEATBALLS**   SERVING SIZE: **4 MEATBALLS**   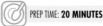 PREP TIME: **20 MINUTES**   COOK TIME: **30 MINUTES**

INGREDIENTS

- ⅓ cup all-natural apricot preserves
- 4½ tsp. **Worcestershire Sauce**
- ¼ tsp. ground ginger
- 3 TB. coconut aminos
- 1 TB. olive oil
- 3 cups green cabbage, thinly chopped
- ¼ cup light coconut milk
- 1½ tsp. tapioca starch
- 1 lb. (450g) ground pork
- ½ lb. (225g) ground veal
- 3 garlic cloves, minced
- 1 tsp. fresh ginger, minced
- ¼ cup green onion, chopped
- 1 TB. coconut oil
- Dash sea salt

METHOD

1 In a small saucepan over medium-high heat, combine apricot preserves, Worcestershire Sauce, ground ginger, and 1 tablespoon coconut aminos. Bring sauce to a boil. Remove from heat, cover, and set aside.

2 Preheat oven to 400°F (200°C).

3 Heat a large skillet over medium-high heat. Add olive oil and cabbage. Sauté for 5 minutes or until cabbage is soft and beginning to brown. Remove from heat.

4 In a large bowl, whisk together coconut milk and tapioca starch.

5 Add cooked cabbage, remaining 2 tablespoons coconut aminos, pork, veal, garlic, ginger, and green onions. With clean hands, mix until well combined.

6 Heat 1 tablespoon coconut oil in a large skillet over high heat. Scoop 1 tablespoon meat mixture and form into a meatball. Place in hot oil and brown on all sides (about 5 minutes). Continue with remaining meat mixture, working in batches.

7 Line a baking sheet with parchment paper. Place browned meatballs on baking sheet and brush with apricot sauce. Bake for 15 minutes or until internal temperature reaches 160°F (70°C). Sprinkle with a dash of sea salt before serving.

Storage: Store meatballs in fridge for up to 1 week or freeze for up to 1 month.

Serving Suggestion: Insert toothpicks and place on a platter as an appetizer or serve over a bed of Cauliflower Fried Rice for an Asian-inspired dinner.

NUTRITION

Calories **309**	Saturated Fat **7g**	Cholesterol **76mg**	Carbohydrate **16g**	Sugar **9g**
Total Fat **18g**	Unsaturated Fat **8g**	Sodium **294mg**	Dietary Fiber **2g**	Protein **21g**

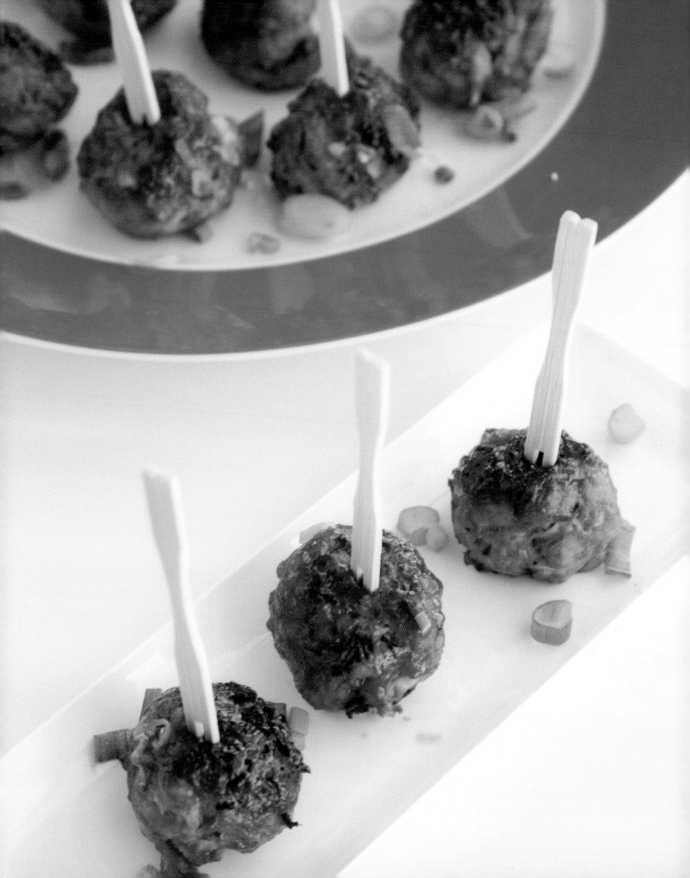

In this refreshing appetizer, **the sweet flavor of fresh shrimp is highlighted with a tangy marinade** of lime juice, vinegar, and creamy avocado.

Citrus Shrimp **Ceviche**

 YIELD: **6 CUPS**   SERVING SIZE: **½ CUP**   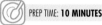 PREP TIME: **10 MINUTES**   CHILL TIME: **I HOUR**

INGREDIENTS

4 cups water

¼ tsp. sea salt

4 limes, halved

1 lb. (450g) shrimp, peeled and deveined

1 cup jicama, peeled and chopped

1 cup green onions, finely chopped

1 tsp. dried oregano

2 tsp. fresh thyme, chopped

¾ cup lime juice

¼ cup apple cider vinegar

1 avocado, chopped

¼ cup cilantro, chopped

¼ tsp. salt

METHOD

1 In a large saucepan over high heat, combine water and salt. Squeeze juice from lime halves into the water and toss in the lime rinds. Bring contents to a boil.

2 Add shrimp and bring contents back to a boil. Remove pan from heat and strain, discarding water and lime rinds.

3 Return hot saucepan to the stovetop and turn off the burner. Place warm shrimp back into the pan, cover, and allow to steam for 5 minutes.

4 Spread shrimp on a baking sheet to cool. Remove tails and chop shrimp into small pieces.

5 In a large bowl, add shrimp, jicama, green onions, oregano, thyme, lime juice, and apple cider vinegar. Refrigerate for 1 hour.

6 Add avocado, cilantro, and salt to taste before serving.

Storage: Ceviche is best served immediately, but can be refrigerated for up to 3 days.

Serving Suggestion: Serve ceviche on top of sliced cucumbers or with crunchy plantain chips.

NUTRITION

Calories 73	Saturated Fat 0g	Cholesterol 0mg	Carbohydrate 7g	Sugar 2g
Total Fat 2g	Unsaturated Fat 0g	Sodium 81mg	Dietary Fiber 2g	Protein 8g

The rich flavors of savory onions and smoky bacon complement the chicken livers featured in this **silky smooth, easy-to-make paté.**

Caramelized **Liverwurst Spread**

 YIELD: **2 CUPS**   SERVING SIZE: **½ CUP**   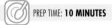 PREP TIME: **10 MINUTES**   COOK TIME: **1 HOUR 30 MIN**

INGREDIENTS

½ lb. (225g) bacon, chopped

2 yellow onions, chopped

2 TB. maple syrup

2 TB. balsamic vinegar

1 bay leaf

¼ cup plus 3 TB. beef broth

2 TB. ghee

1 shallot, finely chopped

1 clove garlic, minced

2 tsp. fresh thyme, chopped

¾ lb. (340g) chicken livers

3 TB. cognac

1 TB. light coconut milk

½ tsp. sea salt

SPECIAL TOOLS

 FOOD PROCESSOR

METHOD

1 In a large skillet over medium-high heat, cook bacon for 10 to 12 minutes or until fat has rendered. Drain all but 1 tablespoon bacon fat.

2 Add onion, maple syrup, balsamic vinegar, bay leaf, and ¼ cup beef broth to skillet. Cover and cook over medium-low heat for 10 minutes or until onions are soft.

3 Remove lid and continue cooking, stirring occasionally, for 60 minutes or until onions are caramelized.

4 Remove bay leaf and transfer to food processor. Pulse to process some, but not all, of the mixture. Transfer to refrigerator.

5 In a large skillet over medium-high heat, heat ghee until melted. Add shallot, garlic, and thyme. Cook for 2 minutes or until soft.

6 Add chicken livers, cognac, and remaining 3 tablespoons beef broth to the skillet. Cook for 5 minutes until livers are browned on the outside and slightly pink on the inside.

7 Remove pan from heat and transfer to clean food processor. Process until smooth. Add coconut milk and sea salt until desired consistency and flavor are obtained.

8 Refrigerate before serving. When ready to serve, fold in the onion-bacon mixture.

Storage: Liver paté is best served immediately.

Serving Suggestion: Serve with plantain chips or chopped veggies.

NUTRITION

Calories 222	Saturated Fat 5g	Cholesterol 161mg	Carbohydrate 12g	Sugar 6g
Total Fat 15g	Unsaturated Fat 5g	Sodium 232mg	Dietary Fiber 2g	Protein 11g

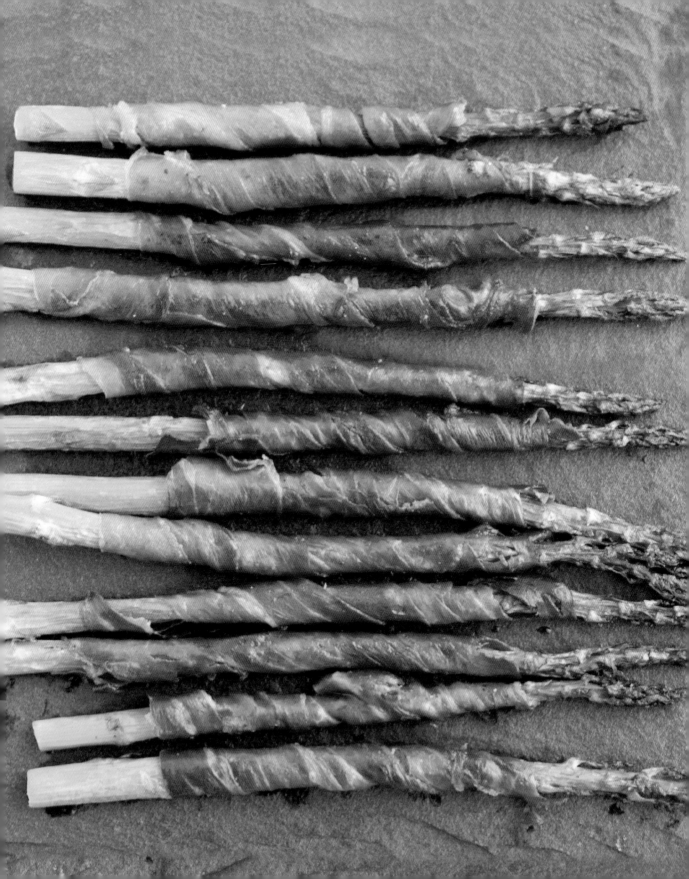

Broiling this easy and elegant finger food creates a **crispy prosciutto** outer layer with a **perfectly tender asparagus** spear inside.

Prosciutto-Wrapped **Asparagus**

 YIELD: **18 SPEARS**   SERVING SIZE: **3 SPEARS**   PREP TIME: **10 MINUTES**   COOK TIME: **10 MINUTES**

INGREDIENTS

18 spears asparagus

1 TB. olive oil

9 pieces prosciutto, cut lengthwise (about 3 oz.; 75g)

METHOD

1 Heat the oven to broil.

2 Trim the woody ends of the asparagus, leaving the heads intact.

3 In a large bowl, toss asparagus spears with olive oil.

4 Wrap each spear with prosciutto, beginning at the head and rolling the prosciutto at a diagonal to allow for minimal overlap of the prosciutto layers.

5 Line a baking sheet with foil. Lay the wrapped asparagus spears on the baking sheet, allowing room between them so they do not touch.

6 Broil for 5 minutes, and then flip the spears and broil for another 5 minutes.

7 Remove the pan from the oven and allow spears to cool slightly before serving.

Serving Suggestion: Prosciutto-Wrapped Asparagus spears are best served immediately to maintain their crispness. This dish can be assembled ahead of time and broiled right before you plan on serving it.

Instead of using a knife, trim the ends of the asparagus by hand. Simply bend each spear until it snaps. The less flexible, dry end will break off, leaving just the moist, tasty part of the spear that you want to eat.

NUTRITION

Calories **60**

Total Fat **4g**

Saturated Fat **1g**

Unsaturated Fat **2g**

Cholesterol **10mg**

Sodium **264mg**

Carbohydrate **2g**

Dietary Fiber **1g**

Sugar **1g**

Protein **5g**

This **homemade savory snack** has the **sweet and salty** flavors you crave without the canola, safflower, or sunflower oil found in most store-bought chips.

Rosemary **Sweet Potato Chips**

 YIELD: **2 CUPS**   SERVING SIZE: **½ CUP**   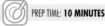 PREP TIME: **10 MINUTES**   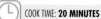 COOK TIME: **20 MINUTES**

INGREDIENTS

2 medium sweet potatoes, peeled

3 TB. olive oil

2 TB. fresh rosemary, finely chopped

¼ tsp. garlic powder

⅛ tsp. sea salt

SPECIAL TOOLS

 MANDOLIN

METHOD

1 Preheat oven to 375°F (190°C). Line a baking sheet with aluminum foil.

2 Using a mandolin or sharp knife, thinly slice sweet potatoes horizontally into ¼-inch (6mm) thick slices.

3 In a large bowl, combine sweet potatoes, olive oil, and rosemary. Toss to coat.

4 Place sweet potato slices on baking sheet and sprinkle with garlic powder and sea salt.

5 Bake for 15 minutes. Reduce heat to 350°F (180°C) and bake for another 5 minutes.

Storage: Store sweet potato chips in an airtight bag or container at room temperature for up to 4 days.

Serving Suggestion: Munch on these chips for a quick snack or dip them in Garlic Herb Avocado Mayo for an easy appetizer.

Variation: Make Thyme Rutabaga Chips by substituting 2 medium rutabaga for the sweet potatoes and 2 tablespoons fresh thyme for the rosemary.

A mandolin will create uniformly sized chips, the key to even cooking. Check on the chips every few minutes and remove the ones that cook more quickly, leaving the remaining chips to continue baking.

NUTRITION

Calories 147

Total Fat 10g

Saturated Fat 1g

Unsaturated Fat 8g

Cholesterol 0mg

Sodium 109mg

Carbohydrate 13g

Dietary Fiber 2g

Sugar 3g

Protein 1g

With only **three ingredients**, these nutrient-dense kale crisps are a **crunchy, salty snack food** you can feel good about eating.

Sea Salt **Kale Crisps**

 YIELD: **6 CUPS**   SERVING SIZE: **1 CUP**   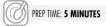 PREP TIME: **5 MINUTES**   COOK TIME: **10 MINUTES**

INGREDIENTS

1 small bunch kale

3 TB. olive oil

Dash sea salt

METHOD

1 Preheat oven to 350°F (180°C). Line a baking sheet with aluminum foil.

2 Remove kale leaves from stems and tear into 2-inch (5cm) pieces.

3 In a large bowl, combine kale and olive oil. Toss to coat, and then massage the oil into each piece of kale.

4 Spread kale evenly in one layer on baking sheet and sprinkle with sea salt.

5 Bake for 10 minutes, flipping the kale chips every 2 minutes.

Storage: Kale chips are best enjoyed immediately, but can be stored in an airtight container at room temperature for up to 48 hours.

Serving Suggestions: Serve alongside Middle Eastern Bison Burgers and Balsamic Grilled Portobello Mushrooms at your next barbecue.

NUTRITION

Calories **127**	Saturated Fat **1g**	Cholesterol **0mg**	Carbohydrate **13g**	Sugar **0g**
Total Fat **8g**	Unsaturated Fat **6g**	Sodium **84mg**	Dietary Fiber **3g**	Protein **4g**

These **crispy chips** are naturally sweet due to the low and slow baking method. The addition of cinnamon creates the perfect combination of **sugar and spice**.

Crispy Cinnamon **Apple Chips**

 YIELD: **ABOUT 30 CHIPS**   SERVING SIZE: **10 CHIPS**   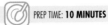 PREP TIME: **10 MINUTES**   COOK TIME: **3–4 HOURS**

INGREDIENTS

3 large Granny Smith or Honeycrisp apples

1 TB. cinnamon

SPECIAL TOOLS

 MANDOLIN

METHOD

1 Preheat oven to 170°F (80°C). Line a baking sheet with parchment paper.

2 Using a mandolin or sharp knife, thinly cut apples horizontally into ¼-inch (.5cm) slices.

3 Lay apple slices on the baking sheet and generously sprinkle with cinnamon.

4 Bake for 3 to 4 hours, until dry and crispy, flipping the apple slices every 30 minutes.

Storage: Store apple chips in an airtight bag or container at room temperature for up to 1 week.

Serving Suggestion: These sweet and spicy apple chips make a perfect snack. Drizzle with Sea Salt Caramel Sauce for a light and healthy dessert to satisfy your sweet tooth.

These apple chips can also be made using a dehydrator. Simply lay the apples on the dehydrator trays, sprinkle generously with cinnamon, and dehydrate at 160°F (70°C) for 6 hours or until crispy.

NUTRITION

| Calories 116 | Saturated Fat 0g | Cholesterol 0mg | Carbohydrate 31g | Sugar 22g |
| Total Fat 0g | Unsaturated Fat 0g | Sodium 3mg | Dietary Fiber 6g | Protein 1g |

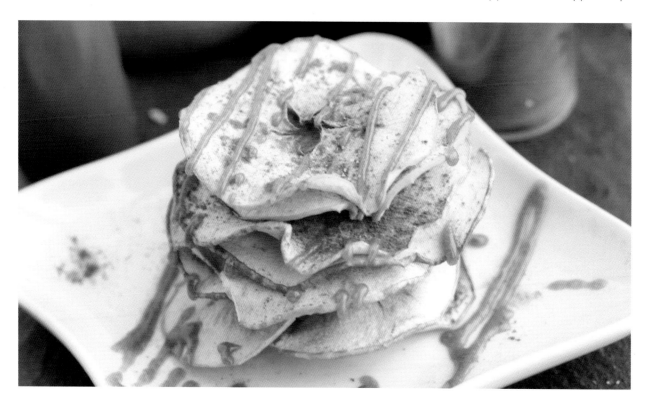

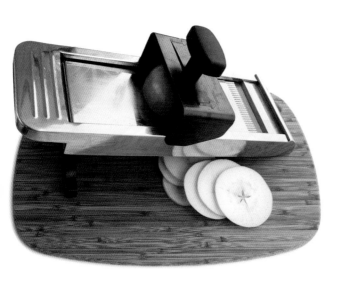

Tips for Using a Mandolin

Safety first. Always use the hand guard when slicing on a mandolin. Firmly attach the fruit or vegetable to the hand guard and begin by slicing slowly and steadily. Using the hand guard will prevent your fingers from accidentally grazing the extremely sharp blade as you slice.

Size matters. Cut fruits and vegetables into manageable pieces (about 4 inches [10cm] long) with smooth, even edges. This will make movement across the blade easy and efficient.

Select the right blade. Most mandolins come with a variety of blades. Select the right blade for the project—use a basic flat blade to cut smooth slices like potato chips, a ridged blade to create a waffle cut, or a julienne blade to create long, thin fries.

This **sweet and refreshing fruit salsa** is perfect for any **summer barbecue** and pairs well with grilled chicken or fish.

Pineapple Mango **Salsa**

 YIELD: **6 CUPS**   SERVING SIZE: ⅓ **CUP**   PREP TIME: **10 MINUTES**   COOK TIME: **30 MINUTES**

INGREDIENTS

2 cups pineapple, chopped

1 cup mango, chopped

1 cup avocado, chopped

½ cup red onion, chopped

2 TB. cilantro, chopped

1 TB. olive oil

2 TB. lime juice

1 TB. honey

Dash sea salt

METHOD

1 In a large bowl, combine pineapple, mango, avocado, red onion, cilantro, olive oil, lime juice, honey, and salt.

2 Refrigerate for at least 30 minutes before serving.

Storage: Store in an airtight container for up to 3 days.

Serving Suggestion: Serve salsa with Rosemary Sweet Potato Chips or scoop on top of Blacked Chicken Breast or Lemon Baked Halibut for a pop of flavor.

NUTRITION

Calories 115	Saturated Fat 1g	Cholesterol 0mg	Carbohydrate 17g	Sugar 12g
Total Fat 6g	Unsaturated Fat 5g	Sodium 29mg	Dietary Fiber 3g	Protein 1g

The **sweetness of parsnip** pairs perfectly with the **spiciness of curry** powder to create a snack that is low in calories and **packed with flavor**.

Curried **Parsnip Ribbons**

 YIELD: **2 CUPS**   SERVING SIZE: ½ **CUP**   PREP TIME: **5 MINUTES**   COOK TIME: **20 MINUTES**

INGREDIENTS

2 parsnips, peeled

1 ½ TB. olive oil

1 ¼ tsp. **Seed-Free Curry Powder**

⅛ tsp. sea salt

METHOD

1 Preheat oven to 400°F (200°C).

2 Using a potato peeler, shave parsnips lengthwise into thin ribbons, making sure to stop peeling when you reach the tough core of the parsnip.

3 In a large bowl, toss parsnip ribbons with olive oil.

4 Line a baking sheet with foil. Spread parsnip ribbons evenly on baking sheet. Bake for 10 minutes until parsnips begin to soften.

5 In a small bowl, combine Seed-Free Curry Powder and salt.

6 Remove parsnips from oven and return to the large bowl. Toss parsnips with spice mixture until well coated.

7 Return parsnip ribbons to baking sheet and bake for another 5 to 10 minutes or until parsnips are golden and crisp.

Storage: Parsnip ribbons are best enjoyed immediately, but can be stored in an airtight container at room temperature for up to 48 hours.

A parsnip is a root vegetable that closely resembles a carrot. With its white color and mild, sweet flavor, this vegetable can be baked, roasted, or puréed into Parsnip Seafood Chowder or Parsnip Purée.

NUTRITION

Calories 97

Total Fat 5g

Saturated Fat 1g

Unsaturated Fat 5g

Cholesterol 0mg

Sodium 80mg

Carbohydrate 13g

Dietary Fiber 3g

Sugar 3g

Protein 1g

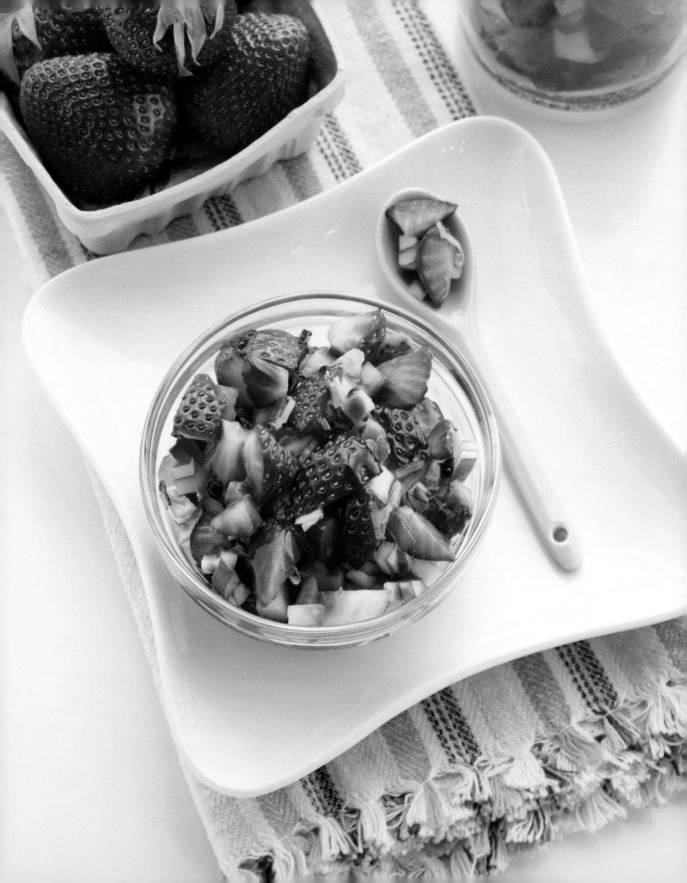

Balsamic vinegar perfectly complements the **strawberries, cherries, and basil** in this **antioxidant-rich salsa**.

Balsamic Strawberry
Basil Salsa

 YIELD: **4 CUPS**   SERVING SIZE: ½ **CUP**   PREP TIME: **10 MINUTES**   COOK TIME: **1 HOUR**

INGREDIENTS

3 cups strawberries, finely chopped

1 cup frozen pitted cherries, finely chopped

½ cup red onion, finely chopped

½ cup fresh basil, chiffonade

1 TB. olive oil

1 TB. balsamic vinegar

METHOD

1 In a large bowl, combine strawberries, cherries, red onion, and basil.

2 Add olive oil and balsamic vinegar and toss to combine.

3 Refrigerate for 1 hour before serving to allow the flavors to meld.

Storage: Store in an airtight container for up to 3 days.

Serving Suggestion: Serve with plantain chips or sliced cucumber for an easy appetizer; scoop on grilled salmon or chicken, or add to your favorite salad for a burst of summertime flavor.

Chiffonade is a chopping technique used to cut delicate herbs into long, thin strips. Stack several basil leaves together and roll them up tightly. Slice perpendicular to the roll.

NUTRITION

| Calories 41 | Saturated Fat 0g | Cholesterol 0mg | Carbohydrate 6g | Sugar 4g |
| Total Fat 2g | Unsaturated Fat 1g | Sodium 1mg | Dietary Fiber 1g | Protein 1g |

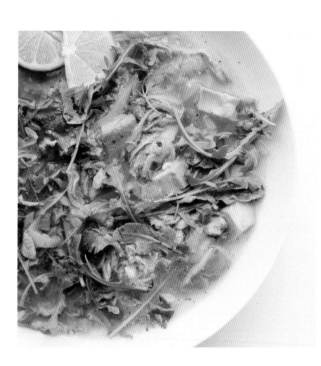

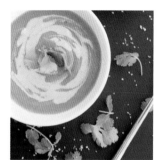

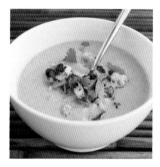

CHAPTER 4

Soups

& Stews

Sweet, caramelized roasted cauliflower is cooked in a rich curry base to create this comforting, Thai-inspired curry cauliflower soup.

Thai **Coconut Curry** Soup

 YIELD: **4 CUPS**   SERVING SIZE: **1 CUP**   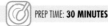 PREP TIME: **30 MINUTES**   COOK TIME: **10 MINUTES**

INGREDIENTS

1 medium head cauliflower, cut into florets

2 TB. coconut oil

2 cups yellow onion, chopped (1 large onion)

Juice and zest from 1 lemon

1 TB. **Seed-Free Curry Powder**

1½ cup vegetable broth

1 (13.5-oz; 400ml) can light coconut milk

½ tsp. honey

¼ tsp. sea salt

1 TB. cilantro, chopped

1 TB. green onions, chopped

SPECIAL TOOLS

 BLENDER

METHOD

1 Preheat oven to 400°F (200°C). Line a baking sheet with foil.

2 Toss cauliflower florets with 1 tablespoon coconut oil and spread on a baking sheet. Bake for 25 minutes or until golden brown.

3 In a large pot or Dutch oven, combine 1 tablespoon coconut oil and onion over medium-high heat. Cook for 3 minutes or until onion begins to soften and become translucent.

4 Add lemon zest, lemon juice, Seed-Free Curry Powder, and ½ cup vegetable broth. Cook for another 2 minutes.

5 Add cauliflower, the remaining vegetable broth, coconut milk, honey, and salt. Stir to combine. Bring mixture to a boil. Remove from heat.

6 Transfer soup to a high-speed blender and blend until smooth.

7 Return soup to pot over low heat and cook until soup begins to thicken (about 2 minutes). Remove from heat and top with cilantro and green onions.

Storage: Store soup in an airtight container in the refrigerator for 1 week or in freezer for up to 3 months.

Serving Suggestion: Serve soup topped with fresh cilantro and green onions or Curried Parsnip Ribbons.

NUTRITION

Calories 189	Saturated Fat 11g	Cholesterol 0mg	Carbohydrate 16g	Sugar 8g
Total Fat 12g	Unsaturated Fat 0g	Sodium 481mg	Dietary Fiber 5g	Protein 4g

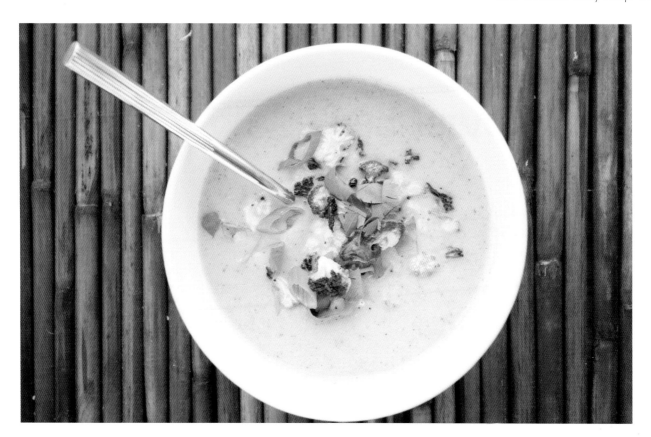

INGREDIENTS: Coconut milk (Filtered Water, Coconut Cream), **Cane Sugar**, Contains 2% or less of: Vitamin & Mineral Blend (Calcium Carbonate, Vitamin A Palmitate, Vitamin B12, Vitamin D2), Sea Salt, Natural Flavor, Sunflower Lecithin, **Guar Gum**, Carrageenan.

Check for ingredients that may irritate the gut.

Avoiding Additives in Store-Bought Coconut Milk

When buying commercially made coconut milk, always be sure to review the list of ingredients on the nutrition label to confirm there is no added sugar or any of the following emulsifiers. While these ingredients can help thicken and stabilize the food, they can also be difficult to digest and irritating to the gut. The simpler the ingredients (i.e., coconut and water), the better.

Guar gum is derived from the starchy endosperm of the guar bean, which is a legume.

Carrageenan comes from a seaweed that goes through extensive processing, including treatment with a chemical alkali solution.

Xanthan gum is a dehydrated byproduct produced by a bacteria grown in a sugar-based solution.

In this **tasty alternative to potato leek soup,** tender roasted cauliflower is puréed into a rich, creamy broth with hints of smoky and tangy flavors.

Cauliflower Leek Soup

 YIELD: **6 CUPS**   SERVING SIZE: **1½ CUP**   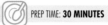 PREP TIME: **30 MINUTES**   COOK TIME: **20 MINUTES**

INGREDIENTS

1 medium head cauliflower, chopped into florets (about 5 cups)

1 TB. coconut oil, melted

1 TB. bacon fat

2 cups leeks, white and light green parts, sliced (about 2 leeks)

3 slices of bacon, chopped

2 cloves garlic, minced

1 TB. fresh thyme, chopped

1 tsp. white wine vinegar

5 cups chicken broth

¼ cup light coconut milk

1 tsp. lemon juice

SPECIAL TOOLS

 BLENDER

METHOD

1 Preheat oven to 400°F (200°C). Line a baking sheet with foil.

2 Place cauliflower on baking sheet and drizzle coconut oil over the cauliflower, massaging it into the florets with clean hands to ensure it is well coated.

3 Bake cauliflower for 15 minutes. Flip cauliflower and bake for another 10 minutes or until crisp and golden brown. Set aside ¼ cup florets for garnish.

4 In a large pot or Dutch oven, heat bacon fat over medium-high heat. Sauté leeks for 10 minutes or until soft and beginning to brown.

5 Add bacon and garlic and cook for another 5 minutes. Add thyme and white wine vinegar and cook for another 2 minutes.

6 Add chicken broth and cooked cauliflower. Bring contents to a boil and then cover and reduce heat. Simmer for 10 minutes. Add coconut milk and lemon juice. Stir to combine.

7 Ladle half of the soup into a high-speed blender. Blend until smooth. Combine blended contents with the remaining soup.

Storage: Store soup in an airtight container in the refrigerator for 1 week or in the freezer for up to 3 months.

Serving Suggestion: Top soup with roasted cauliflower, chopped chives, or bacon bits.

NUTRITION

Calories **165**

Total Fat **11g**

Saturated Fat **6g**

Unsaturated Fat **3g**

Cholesterol **7mg**

Sodium **865mg**

Carbohydrate **14g**

Dietary Fiber **4g**

Sugar **5g**

Protein **5g**

This soup is **bursting with layers of savory, authentic flavor.** You won't even miss the traditional bread and cheese.

French Onion Soup

 YIELD: **4 CUPS**   SERVING SIZE: **1 CUP**   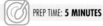 PREP TIME: **5 MINUTES**   COOK TIME: **1 HOUR**

INGREDIENTS

3 yellow onions, thinly sliced (about 4–6 cups)

1 TB. olive oil

¼ tsp. sea salt

1 clove garlic, minced

1 TB. fresh thyme, minced

1 tsp. red wine

1 tsp. white wine vinegar

1 tsp. balsamic vinegar

1 tsp. **Worcestershire Sauce**

4 cups beef broth

METHOD

1 In a large pot or Dutch oven over high heat, combine onions, olive oil, and sea salt.

2 Cook for 30 minutes or until onions are dark and caramelized, stirring frequently and adding a splash of beef broth occasionally to prevent onions from burning.

3 Add garlic and thyme. Cook for another 2 minutes.

4 Add red wine, white wine vinegar, and balsamic vinegar. Cook for another 2 minutes until alcohol has burned off.

5 Add Worcestershire Sauce and beef broth. Bring contents to a boil. Reduce heat to low and simmer, partially covered for 25 minutes.

Storage: Store soup in an airtight container in the refrigerator for 1 week or in the freezer for up to 3 months.

Serving Suggestion: Stir in some chopped Greek-Style Roast Chicken, Sunday Slow Cooker Pot Roast, or Orange Pulled Pork Carnitas for added protein.

NUTRITION

Calories **159**

Total Fat **3g**

Saturated Fat **0g**

Unsaturated Fat **2g**

Cholesterol **0mg**

Sodium **749mg**

Carbohydrate **8g**

Dietary Fiber **5g**

Sugar **0g**

Protein **3g**

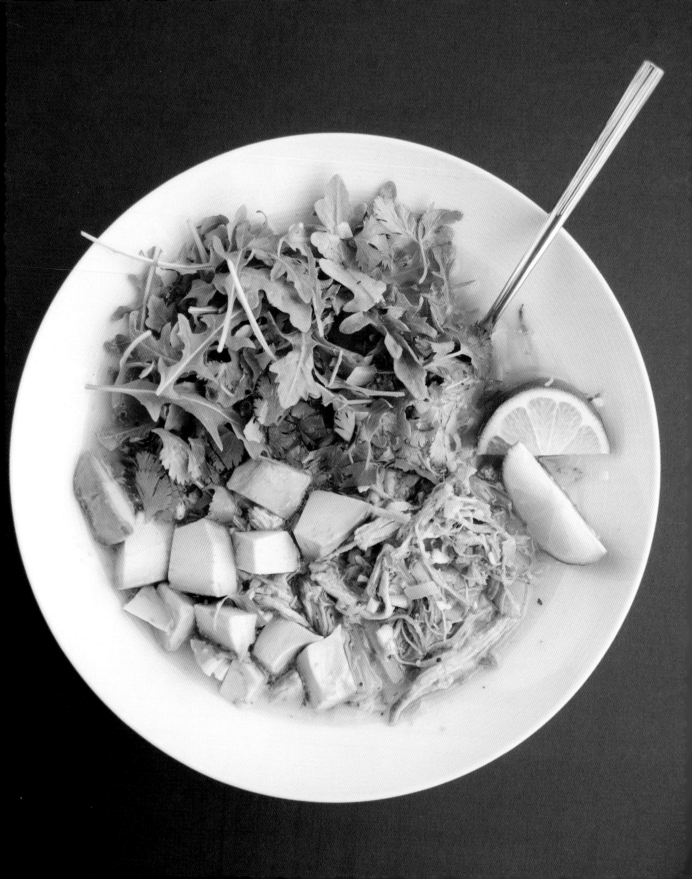

Savor the rich flavors of **slow-cooked shredded pork and garlic** with the freshness of lime, cilantro, arugula, and avocado.

Mexican Carnitas
Broth Bowl

 YIELD: **6 CUPS**   SERVING SIZE: **1 CUP**   PREP TIME: **10 MINUTES**   COOK TIME: **40 MINUTES**

INGREDIENTS

2 TB. olive oil

2 cups white onion, chopped (1 large onion)

1 cup chayote squash, peeled, core removed, and chopped (1 medium squash)

6 garlic cloves, minced

4 cups chicken broth

3 cups **Orange Pulled Pork Carnitas**

3 TB. lime juice

Dash sea salt

2 cups arugula

½ cup cilantro

1 avocado, chopped

METHOD

1 In a large pot or Dutch oven, heat olive oil, onion, and chayote over medium-high heat. Sauté for 5 minutes or until vegetables are soft.

2 Add garlic and sauté for another 2 minutes until fragrant.

3 Add chicken broth and Orange Pulled Pork Carnitas. Bring to a boil. Reduce heat, cover, and simmer for 30 minutes.

4 Stir in lime juice and salt. When ready to serve, ladle soup into bowls, top with arugula, cilantro, and avocado.

Storage: Store carnitas broth separate from arugula, cilantro, and avocado. When ready to enjoy, stir the fresh ingredients into the hot broth. Refrigerate soup for up to 1 week or freeze for up to 3 months.

Originally from Mexico, chayote squash is now enjoyed in many cultures. It has white flesh, a crisp texture, and a mild sweet flavor. Cook it like summer squash, or enjoy it raw in salads or salsas.

NUTRITION

Calories **455**	Saturated Fat **10g**	Cholesterol **94mg**	Carbohydrate **9g**	Sugar **2g**
Total Fat **36g**	Unsaturated Fat **23g**	Sodium **547mg**	Dietary Fiber **4g**	Protein **24g**

This hearty chowder is loaded with rich, creamy flavor, thanks to four different types of seafood and sweet, earthy parsnips.

Parsnip Seafood Chowder

 YIELD: **8 CUPS**   SERVING SIZE: **1 CUP**   PREP TIME: **20 MINUTES**   COOK TIME: **30 MINUTES**

INGREDIENTS

2 TB. olive oil

1 TB. ghee

2 cups yellow onion, chopped

1 cup celery, chopped

3 cups parsnips, peeled and chopped

2 TB. fresh thyme

1 bay leaf

1 cup clam juice

½ cup water

½ cup vegetable broth

1½ cup light coconut milk

½ lb. (225g) peeled and deveined shrimp, chopped

½ lb. (225g) bay scallops, chopped

½ lb. (225g) monkfish (or other mild white fish)

½ lb. (225g) crab meat

1 tsp. lemon juice

¼ cup parsley, chopped

METHOD

1 In a large pot or Dutch oven, heat olive oil and ghee over medium-high heat.

2 Add onion, celery, and parsnips. Cook for 10 minutes. Add thyme and continue cooking for another 5 minutes or until vegetables are soft.

2 Add bay leaf, clam juice, water, broth, and coconut milk. Bring to a boil.

3 Reduce heat and add shrimp, scallops, monkfish, and crab meat. Simmer on low for 10 minutes or until fish is cooked through.

4 Transfer 2 cups of soup to a high-speed blender. Blend until smooth. Return purée back to pot and combine with remaining soup. Stir in lemon juice and parsley.

Storage: Store soup in an airtight container in the refrigerator for 1 week or in the freezer for up to 3 months.

> When blending hot soups, remove the plastic stopper from the blender lid and cover the opening with a dish towel to allow steam to escape.

NUTRITION

Calories 286

Total Fat 12g

Saturated Fat 2g

Unsaturated Fat 6g

Cholesterol 61mg

Sodium 471mg

Carbohydrate 15g

Dietary Fiber 4g

Sugar 4g

Protein 24g

SPECIAL TOOLS

 BLENDER

Cooking the mushrooms low and slow creates a meaty texture that pairs perfectly with the **deep flavors of beef broth and pork meatballs**.

Wild Mushroom
Meatball Stew

 YIELD: **6 CUPS**   SERVING SIZE: **1 CUP**   PREP TIME: **10 MINUTES**   COOK TIME: **1 HOUR**

INGREDIENTS

8 cups mushrooms, chopped

2 cups onion, chopped

2 garlic cloves, minced

2 TB. fresh thyme, chopped

4 TB. ghee

4 cups beef broth

12 mini **Pork and Fennel Meatballs**

¼ cup parsley, chopped

SPECIAL TOOLS

 BLENDER

METHOD

1 In a large pot or Dutch oven over medium-high heat, combine mushrooms, onion, garlic, thyme, and ghee.

2 Cook for 30 minutes, stirring occasionally until mushrooms have released all of their liquid and begin to caramelize.

3 Add beef broth and bring to a boil. Reduce heat, cover, and simmer for 20 minutes.

4 Ladle 1 cup of the soup into blender and blend until smooth. Return puréed soup to pot and combine with remaining soup.

5 Add meatballs and bring soup to a boil. Remove from heat and stir in parsley.

Storage: Store soup in an airtight container in the refrigerator for 1 week or in the freezer for up to 3 months.

NUTRITION

| Calories 240 | Saturated Fat 9g | Cholesterol 43mg | Carbohydrate 10g | Sugar 4g |
| Total Fat 19g | Unsaturated Fat 9g | Sodium 439mg | Dietary Fiber 3g | Protein 9g |

The **fresh flavors of asparagus and broccoli** are highlighted by smoky bacon and creamy coconut milk in this savory spring soup.

Spring Asparagus and
Broccoli Bisque

 YIELD: **4 CUPS**   SERVING SIZE: **1 CUP**   PREP TIME: **20 MINUTES**   COOK TIME: **15 MINUTES**

INGREDIENTS

1 lb. (450g) asparagus, ends trimmed

3 cups broccoli florets

1 TB. olive oil

⅛ tsp. sea salt

1 TB. bacon fat

½ cup shallot, chopped

2 cloves garlic, minced

2 cups vegetable broth

1 cup light coconut milk

2 TB. lemon juice

SPECIAL TOOLS

 BLENDER

METHOD

1 Preheat oven to 375°F (190°C). Line a baking sheet with foil.

2 Place asparagus and broccoli on baking sheet. Drizzle with olive oil and massage oil into vegetables until coated. Sprinkle with sea salt. Roast vegetables for 20 minutes.

3 In a large pot or Dutch oven, heat bacon fat over medium-high heat. Add shallots and garlic. Cook for 5 minutes or until soft.

4 Add vegetable broth, coconut milk, and lemon juice. Bring contents to a boil. Remove pan from heat.

5 In a blender, combine asparagus, broccoli, and broth. Blend for 30 seconds or until smooth.

6 Return soup to pot and warm over low heat before serving.

Storage: Store soup in an airtight container in the refrigerator for 1 week or in the freezer for up to 3 months.

NUTRITION

Calories **164**	Saturated Fat **2g**	Cholesterol **3mg**	Carbohydrate **17g**	Sugar **5g**
Total Fat **10g**	Unsaturated Fat **5g**	Sodium **393mg**	Dietary Fiber **6g**	Protein **5g**

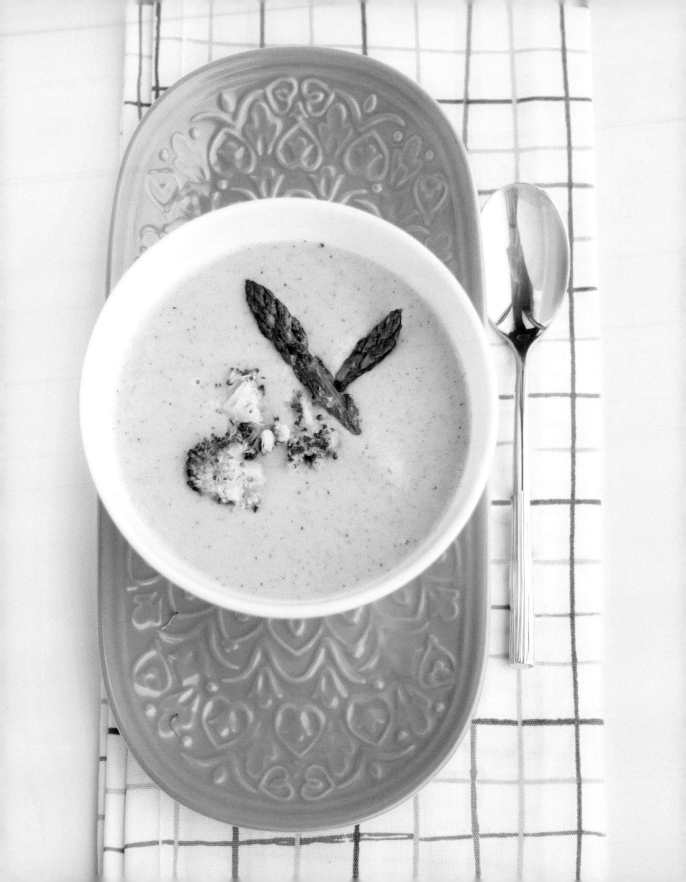

This AIP-friendly version of the traditional Italian favorite has **warm winter soup flavors of oregano and basil** with loads of nutritious, fibrous veggies.

Hearty
Minestrone Soup

 YIELD: **6 CUPS**   SERVING SIZE: **1 CUP**   PREP TIME: **10 MINUTES**   COOK TIME: **30 MINUTES**

INGREDIENTS

2 TB. olive oil

2 cups yellow onion, chopped (1 large onion)

1 cup carrot, peeled and chopped (2 large carrots)

1 cup celery, chopped (1 large celery stalk)

4 cloves garlic, minced

1 tsp. dried oregano

1 tsp. dried basil

½ tsp. garlic powder

1 bay leaf

¼ cup **Tomato-Less Pasta Sauce**

4 cups vegetable broth

1 cup water

2 cups kale, stems removed and chopped

1 cup frozen green beans, halved

1½ cup zucchini, chopped

METHOD

1 Heat a large pot or Dutch oven over medium-high heat.

2 Add oil, onion, carrot, celery, and garlic. Sauté for 5 minutes or until they begin to soften.

3 Add the oregano, basil, garlic powder, bay leaf, and Tomato-Less Pasta Sauce. Cook for another 2 minutes.

4 Add vegetable broth and water. Bring to a boil and then reduce heat, cover, and simmer for 10 minutes.

5 Add kale, green beans, and zucchini. Cover and continue to simmer for another 10 minutes.

Storage: Store soup in an airtight container in the refrigerator for 1 week, or in freezer for up to 3 months.

Serving Suggestion: Serve warm and top with fresh chopped basil. Serve with a green salad for a quick and easy lunch.

NUTRITION

Calories 119

Total Fat 5g

Saturated Fat 1g

Unsaturated Fat 5g

Cholesterol 0mg

Sodium 475mg

Carbohydrate 16g

Dietary Fiber 3g

Sugar 6g

Protein 3g

Coconut milk and pancetta give this winter classic a **creamy texture and savory flavor** that will warm your stomach on even the coldest of days.

Classic **Chicken and Cauliflower** Rice Soup

 YIELD: **6 CUPS**   SERVING SIZE: **1 CUP**   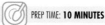 PREP TIME: **10 MINUTES**   COOK TIME: **30 MINUTES**

INGREDIENTS

4oz. (110g) pancetta, chopped (¼ cup)

2 cups yellow onion, chopped (1 large onion)

1 cup carrot, peeled and chopped (2 large carrots)

1 cup celery, chopped (1 large celery stalk)

4 cloves garlic, minced

1 TB. fresh thyme, chopped

1 TB. fresh rosemary, chopped

4 cups chicken broth

1 cup light coconut milk

2 TB. tapioca starch

2 cups cooked chicken, chopped

2 cups cauliflower, riced

METHOD

1 Heat a large pot or Dutch oven over medium-high heat. Add pancetta and cook for 5 minutes or until crisp.

2 Add onion, carrot, celery, and garlic to the pancetta. Sauté for 5 minutes or until veggies begin to soften.

3 Add thyme, rosemary, and chicken broth and bring contents to a boil.

4 In a small bowl, whisk together coconut milk and tapioca starch.

5 Add chicken, cauliflower, and coconut milk mixture to pot. Stir to combine.

6 Bring contents back to a boil. Reduce heat and simmer uncovered for 10 minutes.

Storage: Store in an airtight container in the refrigerator for 1 week, or in freezer for up to 3 months.

Serving Suggestion: Serve warm and top with fresh chopped parsley.

NUTRITION

Calories 210

Total Fat 8g

Saturated Fat 4g

Unsaturated Fat 0g

Cholesterol 30mg

Sodium 357mg

Carbohydrate 15g

Dietary Fiber 3g

Sugar 5g

Protein 19g

This healthy and rustic stew features **hearty bites of sweet butternut squash,** savory pork sausage, and crunchy kale.

Tuscan **Sausage and Kale** Stew

 YIELD: **4 CUPS**   SERVING SIZE: **1 CUP**   PREP TIME: **5 MINUTES**   COOK TIME: **40 MINUTES**

INGREDIENTS

1 TB. olive oil

½ lb. (225g) pork sausage, sliced

2 cups white onion, chopped (1 large onion)

2 cloves garlic, minced

1 cup butternut squash, peeled and chopped

2 bay leaves

1 tsp. dried oregano

4 cups chicken broth

¼ cup canned sweet potato purée

2 cups kale, stems removed and chopped

METHOD

1 In a large pot or Dutch oven, heat olive oil over medium-high heat. Add sausage, onion, and garlic. Cook for 5 minutes or until meat is no longer pink and vegetables are soft.

2 Add butternut squash and cook for another 10 minutes until vegetables are caramelized and sausage is golden brown.

3 Add bay leaves, oregano, and chicken broth. Bring to a boil.

4 Reduce heat and cover. Simmer stew for 30 minutes.

5 Stir in sweet potato purée and kale. Cook for another 5 minutes or until kale is slightly wilted.

Storage: Store soup in an airtight container in the refrigerator for 1 week or in the freezer for up to 3 months.

NUTRITION

| Calories 245 | Saturated Fat 4g | Cholesterol 24mg | Carbohydrate 18g | Sugar 3g |
| Total Fat 15g | Unsaturated Fat 9g | Sodium 1,084mg | Dietary Fiber 1g | Protein 9g |

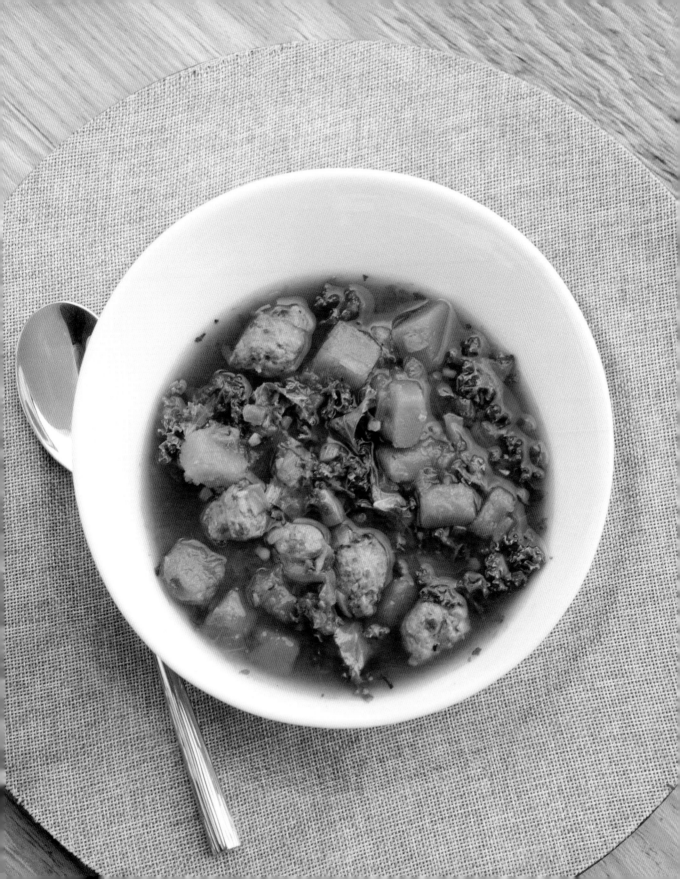

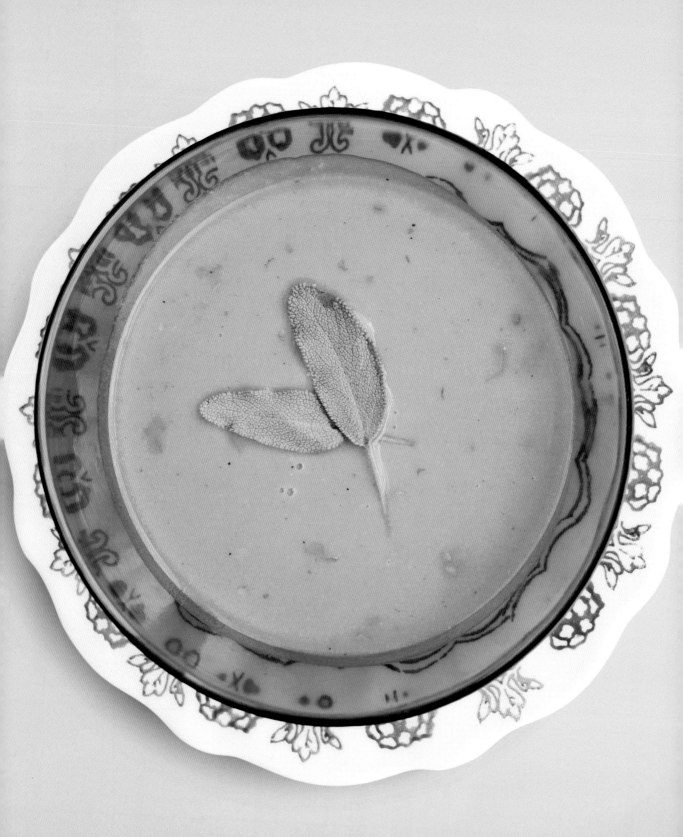

In this **elegant autumn soup,** hearty roasted butternut squash is puréed and paired with a subtle sage cream.

Roasted **Butternut Squash and Sage** Soup

 YIELD: **6 CUPS**   SERVING SIZE: **1 CUP**   PREP TIME: **10 MINUTES**   COOK TIME: **30 MINUTES**

INGREDIENTS

6 cups butternut squash, peeled and cubed

2 TB. olive oil

⅛ tsp. sea salt

1 cup light coconut milk

3 TB. fresh sage, chopped

2 TB. ghee

1 cup shallots, chopped

2 garlic cloves, minced

4 cups **Bone Broth** (or chicken broth)

SPECIAL TOOLS

 BLENDER

METHOD

1 Preheat oven to 400°F (200°C). Line a baking sheet with foil. Spread butternut squash on baking sheet, massage with olive oil, and sprinkle with sea salt.

2 Roast squash for 15 minutes. Turn squash, and bake for another 15 minutes. Remove from oven and set aside.

3 In a large pot or Dutch oven, heat coconut milk over medium-high heat. Add sage and stir. Bring to a boil. Transfer contents into a small bowl and set aside for 10 minutes to steep.

4 In a clean pot or Dutch oven, heat ghee over medium-high heat. Add shallots and garlic. Cook for 2 to 3 minutes or until soft.

5 Add roasted butternut squash and Bone Broth. Bring contents to a boil. Reduce heat and simmer, covered, for 10 minutes.

6 Transfer contents to a high-speed blender. Blend contents until smooth.

7 Return soup to pot and stir in the coconut milk and sage mixture.

Storage: Store soup in an airtight container in the refrigerator for 1 week or in the freezer for up to 3 months.

Variation: To make **Spiced Carrot Soup,** replace butternut squash with chopped carrots and replace sage with fresh grated ginger.

NUTRITION

Calories 240

Total Fat 13g

Saturated Fat 4g

Unsaturated Fat 6g

Cholesterol 16mg

Sodium 88mg

Carbohydrate 23g

Dietary Fiber 5g

Sugar 4g

Protein 7g

This hearty puréed soup is **topped with a tangy garlic herb chermoula sauce**, a classic Moroccan sauce traditionally used to top fish and chicken.

Moroccan **Sweet Potato** Soup

 YIELD: **6 CUPS**   SERVING SIZE: **1 CUP**   PREP TIME: **10 MINUTES**   COOK TIME: **30 MINUTES**

INGREDIENTS

- 2 TB. olive oil
- 2 cups yellow onion, chopped (1 large onion)
- 2 cups sweet potato, peeled and chopped (1 medium potato)
- 2 cups parsnips, peeled and chopped (2–3 medium parsnips)
- 1 cup carrots, peeled and chopped (2–3 medium carrots)
- 1 TB. fresh ginger, peeled and minced
- 9 cloves garlic, minced
- 1 TB. **Seed-Free Curry Powder**
- 4 cups vegetable broth
- Juice of 2 lemons
- ½ cup cilantro, leaves and stems, chopped
- ½ cup parsley
- ¼ cup coconut milk

SPECIAL TOOLS

 BLENDER

METHOD

1. Heat olive oil in large pot or Dutch oven over medium-high heat.

2. Add onion, sweet potato, parsnips, carrots, ginger, and 3 teaspoons minced garlic. Sauté for 5 minutes or until onion begins to soften.

3. Add Seed-Free Curry Powder and ½ cup broth. Cook for another 2 minutes until fragrant.

4. Add remaining 3½ cups vegetable broth and bring contents to a boil. Reduce heat to low, cover, and simmer for 30 minutes.

5. Remove from heat and transfer contents to a blender. Blend on high until smooth. Return soup to pot.

6. In a clean blender, combine remaining minced garlic, lemon juice, cilantro, parsley, and coconut milk to make chermoula sauce. Blend until smooth.

7. Stir 1 tablespoon chermoula sauce into each serving of soup.

Storage: Store soup and chermoula sauce separately in the refrigerator for up to 1 week or in the freezer up to 3 months.

Serving Suggestion: Serve soup topped with chermoula sauce and additional fresh cilantro.

NUTRITION

Calories 155
Total Fat 7g
Saturated Fat 2g
Unsaturated Fat 4g
Cholesterol 0mg
Sodium 429mg
Carbohydrate 22g
Dietary Fiber 4g
Sugar 5g
Protein 2g

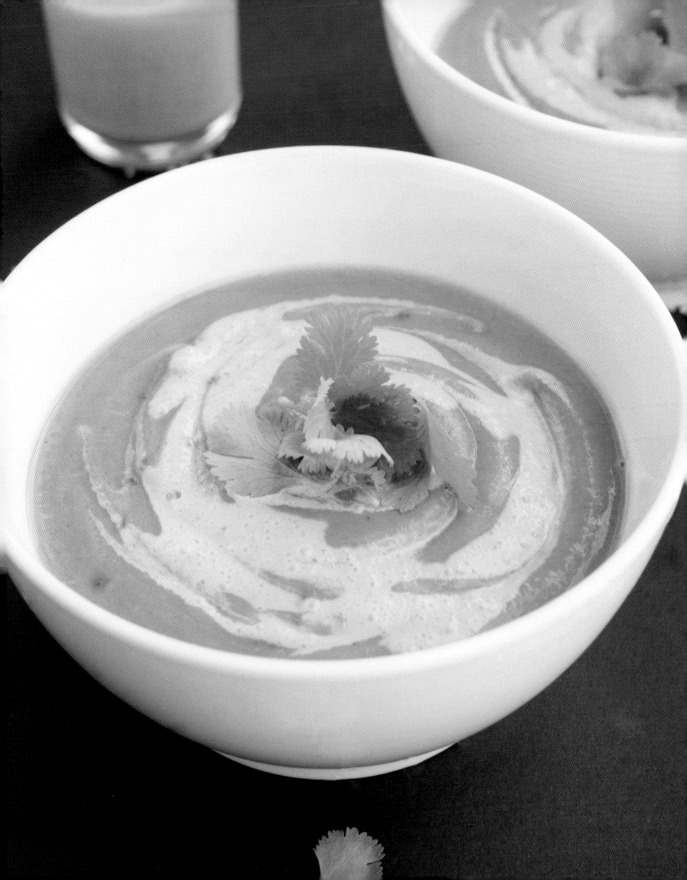

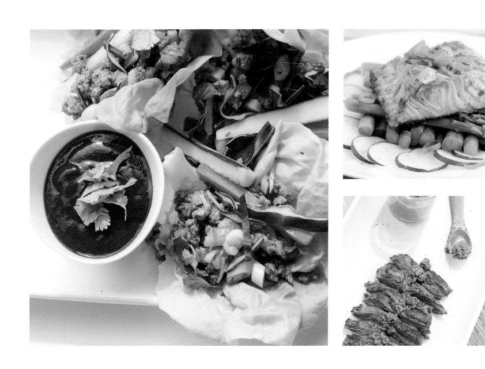

CHAPTER 5

Main Courses

With flavors of ginger and orange zest, a quick and easy marinade gives this **omega-3 rich salmon** a sweet, tangy citrus glaze.

Honey Ginger
Glazed Salmon

 4 FILETS   **1 FILET**   **1 HOUR**   **15 MINUTES**

INGREDIENTS

- ¼ cup orange juice
- ¼ cup honey
- ¼ cup coconut aminos
- 1 TB. olive oil
- 1 cup green onions, sliced (4 green onions)
- 1 TB. fresh ginger, peeled
- 1 TB. sherry vinegar
- ½ tsp orange zest
- 4 (4-oz.; 112g) salmon filets, skin on

METHOD

1 In a food processor, combine orange juice, honey, coconut aminos, olive oil, ½ cup green onions, ginger, sherry vinegar, and orange zest. Process for 30 seconds or until well combined.

2 Pour marinade into a zipper-lock plastic bag. Add salmon and seal. Refrigerate and marinate salmon for 1 hour.

3 Heat a medium skillet over medium-high heat. Add salmon to hot pan, skin side down. Spoon ¼ cup marinade over the salmon. Allow to cook for 3 minutes.

4 Flip salmon and cook for another 3 minutes or until salmon is flaky and cooked through.

Storage: Salmon is best served immediately, but leftovers can be refrigerated and used for lunch or dinner the following day.

Serving Suggestion: Serve salmon over leafy greens or vegetable of your choice and garnish with sliced green onions.

SPECIAL TOOLS

 FOOD PROCESSOR

NUTRITION

Calories 249
Total Fat 7g
Saturated Fat 1g
Unsaturated Fat 6g
Cholesterol 59mg
Sodium 412mg
Carbohydrate 22g
Dietary Fiber 0g
Sugar 19g
Protein 23g

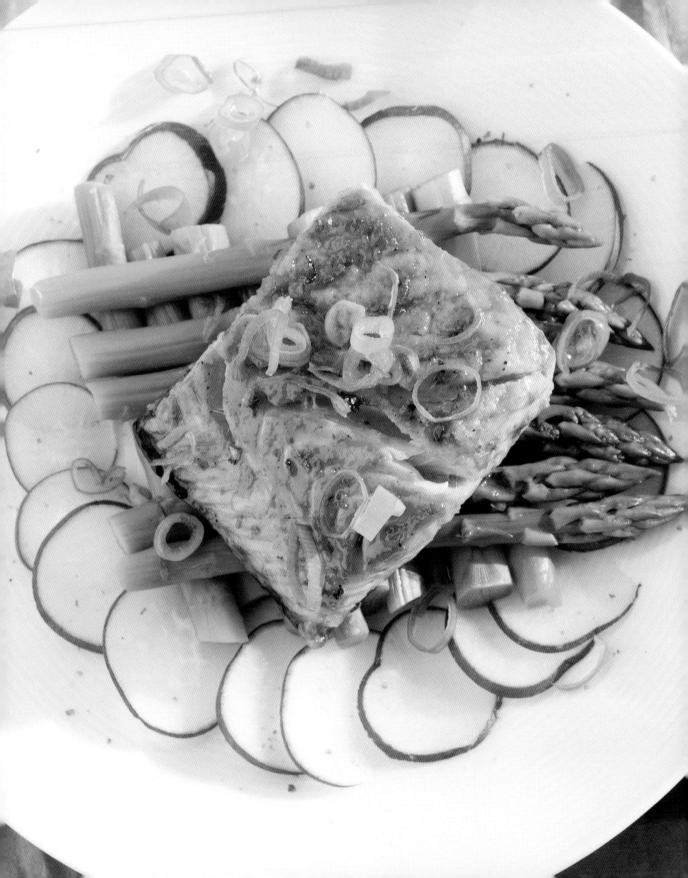

This garlic-infused pot roast becomes deliciously tender in the slow cooker. With a tangy shallot sauce, it's **comfort food at its best.**

Sunday Slow Cooker **Pot Roast**

 YIELD: **8 SLICES**   SERVING SIZE: **1 SLICE**   PREP TIME: **10 MINUTES**   COOK TIME: **7 HOURS**

INGREDIENTS

2 cups parsnips, peeled and chopped (3–4 parsnips)

2 cups sweet potatoes, peeled and chopped (1 large sweet potato)

2 cups shallots, chopped

3 lb. (1.5kg) boneless chuck roast

8 cloves garlic, thinly sliced

1½ tsp. sea salt

1½ cups beef broth

2 TB. **Worcestershire Sauce**

2 tsp. lemon juice

¼ cup ghee, melted

1 TB. tapioca starch

½ cup parsley, chopped

SPECIAL TOOLS

 SLOW COOKER

METHOD

1 Place parsnips, sweet potatoes, and shallots at the bottom of a slow cooker.

2 Using a paring knife, make small cuts into both sides of the chuck roast. Insert garlic slices into the cuts and season chuck roast with 1 teaspoon sea salt

3 Put seasoned chuck roast into slow cooker, nestling it among the vegetables.

4 In a small bowl, whisk together beef broth, Worcestershire Sauce, lemon juice, and remaining ½ teaspoon sea salt. Pour sauce into slow cooker over chuck roast.

5 Cover and cook meat and vegetables in slow cooker on low for 7 hours.

6 Remove roast and vegetables from the slow cooker with a slotted spoon.

7 In a small bowl, whisk together ghee, tapioca starch, and parsley. Add contents to the juices in the slow cooker and stir to combine.

8 Slice pot roast and spoon slow cooker sauce over meat and vegetables.

Storage: Refrigerate pot roast for 5 days or freeze for up to 3 months.

Serving Suggestion: Serve sliced pot roast over vegetables and spoon sauce over the top before serving.

NUTRITION

Calories 369

Total Fat 22g

Saturated Fat 4g

Unsaturated Fat 8g

Cholesterol 74mg

Sodium 726mg

Carbohydrate 23g

Dietary Fiber 3g

Sugar 4g

Protein 18g

Beef and broccoli are coated with a **sweet-and-salty ginger garlic sauce** in this dish that mimics familiar restaurant-style flavors.

Broccoli Beef Stir-Fry

 YIELD: **4 CUPS**   SERVING SIZE: **1 CUP**   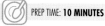 PREP TIME: **10 MINUTES**   COOK TIME: **20 MINUTES**

INGREDIENTS

1 TB. olive oil

1 cup yellow onion, chopped (½ large onion)

1 lb. (450g) flank steak, thinly sliced

¼ cup water

4 cups broccoli, chopped (½ large broccoli head)

½ cup coconut aminos

½ cup beef broth

5 garlic cloves, minced

1 tsp. fresh ginger, minced

2 TB. fish sauce

1 tsp. honey

1 tsp. tapioca starch

METHOD

1 Heat olive oil in a large skillet over medium-high heat. Add onion and cook for 5 minutes or until soft and translucent.

2 Add flank steak and cook for 5 minutes, flipping occasionally to brown on both sides.

3 Remove steak and onions from skillet and set aside. Add water and broccoli.

4 Cover and steam for 3 minutes until soft. Remove broccoli from pan.

5 In a small bowl, whisk together coconut aminos, beef broth, garlic, ginger, fish sauce, honey, and tapioca starch.

6 Add sauce to skillet and whisk over medium heat until bubbling and beginning to thicken. Return meat and broccoli to pan and toss to coat.

Storage: Refrigerate for up to 5 days.

Serving Suggestion: Serve over Cauliflower Fried Rice and top with chopped green onions.

NUTRITION

Calories 313

Total Fat 16g

Saturated Fat 8g

Unsaturated Fat 1g

Cholesterol 49mg

Sodium 890mg

Carbohydrate 18g

Dietary Fiber 3g

Sugar 4g

Protein 24g

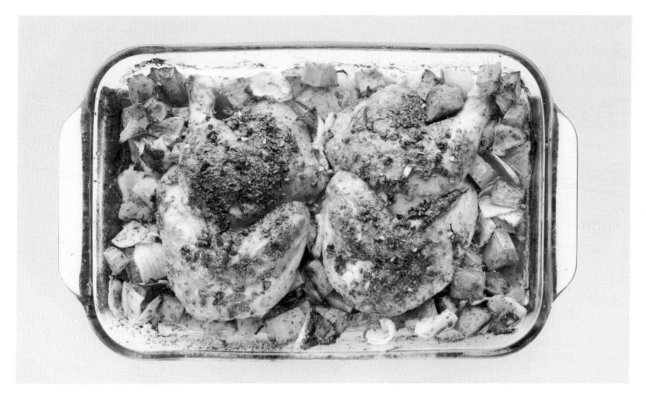

Repurpose Leftover Chicken

Any leftover meat can be saved to use for other meals. Just remove it from the bones and refrigerate until needed.

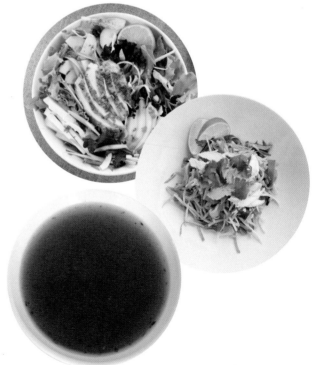

Salads: Sliced, chopped, or shredded grilled chicken is perfect for topping your favorite salad. Use leftover chicken to make Avocado Chicken Salad.

Soups & Stews: Use leftover cooked chicken in a soup or stew, like Classic Chicken and Cauliflower Rice Soup, for added protein and flavor.

Bone Broth: Save your roast chicken bones in the freezer until you have enough for a batch of Bone Broth.

This traditional Greek-style roast chicken is **coated in savory olive oil and tangy lemon juice** and generously sprinkled with flavorful oregano.

Greek-Style **Roast Chicken**

 YIELD: **8 PIECES**   SERVING SIZE: **1 PIECE**   PREP TIME: **20 MINUTES**   COOK TIME: **1 HOUR 20 MIN**

INGREDIENTS

1 (4.5-lb; 2.1kg) roasting chicken, without giblets

Juice of 3 lemons

½ cup olive oil

¼ tsp. sea salt

¼ tsp. garlic powder

¼ tsp. onion powder

2 TB. dried oregano

10 cloves garlic, minced

1 large yellow onion, quartered

2 medium sweet potatoes, cubed

METHOD

1 Preheat oven to 375°F (190°C). Line the bottom of a baking dish with parchment paper.

2 Rinse chicken under cold water and pat dry with paper towels. Using a sharp knife or poultry shears, cut chicken in half along the backbone. Discard the backbone and lay the two chicken halves on the parchment paper.

3 Pour the lemon juice over the chicken halves, rubbing it into the skin.

4 Drizzle ¼ cup olive oil over the chicken, massaging it into the chicken.

5 In a small bowl, combine salt, garlic powder, onion powder, and oregano.

6 Season chicken halves with half of the seasoning mixture.

7 In a large bowl, combine garlic, onion, sweet potatoes, remaining ¼ cup olive oil, and remaining half of seasoning mixture. Toss to combine. Spread onion and sweet potatoes mixture around the chicken halves.

8 Bake uncovered for 1 hour and 20 minutes, basting occasionally with juices from the bottom of the pan keep chicken moist.

Storage: Store in refrigerator for up to 1 week or in freezer for up to 3 months.

NUTRITION

Calories 624

Total Fat 41g

Saturated Fat 10g

Unsaturated Fat 15g

Cholesterol 214mg

Sodium 241mg

Carbohydrate 14g

Dietary Fiber 3g

Sugar 3g

Protein 51g

These pan-fried pork chops are **coated in a glossy apple cider glaze and seared to perfection** with the sweet autumn flavors of apple and cinnamon.

Apple Cider **Pork Chops**

 YIELD: **4 PORK CHOPS**   SERVING SIZE: **1 PORK CHOP**   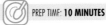 PREP TIME: **10 MINUTES**   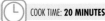 COOK TIME: **20 MINUTES**

INGREDIENTS

1½ cup unsweetened apple juice

¼ cup pure maple syrup

2 TB. **Worcestershire Sauce**

⅛ tsp. cinnamon

4 (4-oz.; 110g) pork chops, bone in with fat

⅛ tsp sea salt 1 TB. olive oil

1 apple, cored and chopped

1 tsp. fresh thyme, chopped

SPECIAL TOOLS

 MEAT THERMOMETER

METHOD

1 To make apple cider sauce, combine apple juice, maple syrup, Worcestershire Sauce, and cinnamon in a small saucepan. Bring contents to a boil. Reduce heat, cover, and simmer for 10 minutes. Remove from heat and set aside.

2 Heat olive oil in skillet over medium-high heat. Season both sides of pork chops with sea salt. Add pork chops and spoon ½ cup apple cider sauce on top.

3 Cook pork chops for 5 minutes per side or until internal temperature reaches 145°F (65°C), spooning sauce over pork chops occasionally to prevent pan from burning. Remove pork chops from heat and set aside.

4 Add chopped apple to pan with remaining sauce. Bring contents to a boil. Reduce heat and simmer for 10 minutes or until sauce has reduced by at least half.

5 Place pork chops on serving platter, top with apple and sauce mixture, and garnish with fresh thyme.

Storage: Pork chops can be refrigerated for up to 4 days.

NUTRITION

Calories **300**

Total Fat **8g**

Saturated Fat **2g**

Unsaturated Fat **2g**

Cholesterol **78mg**

Sodium **331mg**

Carbohydrate **31g**

Dietary Fiber **1g**

Sugar **29g**

Protein **26g**

This AIP version of the classic Catalan romesco sauce features **savory garlic and sweet carrots,** which pair nicely with the spiciness of arugula.

Pork Tenderloin
with Roasted Carrot Romesco

 YIELD: **8 (2-OZ.; 55G) SLICES**   SERVING SIZE: **2 SLICES**   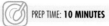 PREP TIME: **10 MINUTES**   COOK TIME: **20 MINUTES**

INGREDIENTS

- 1½ lb. (680g) small carrots, peeled and halved lengthwise
- 3 TB. olive oil
- ¼ tsp. sea salt
- 1 lb. (450g) boneless pork tenderloin
- 1 clove garlic, peeled
- 2 TB. red wine vinegar
- 2 cups arugula

SPECIAL TOOLS

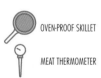

OVEN-PROOF SKILLET

MEAT THERMOMETER

FOOD PROCESSOR

METHOD

1 Preheat oven to 450°F (230°C). Line a baking sheet with foil.

2 Toss carrots with 1 tablespoon olive oil and ⅛ teaspoon sea salt. Lay carrots on baking sheet and roast for 15 to 20 minutes, turning occasionally until soft. Remove pan from oven and set aside.

3 In a large, oven-proof skillet, heat 1 tablespoon olive oil over medium-high heat. Season pork with ⅛ teaspoon sea salt. Cook pork in pan, turning occasionally, for 10 to 15 minutes, until golden brown on all sides.

4 Transfer skillet to oven and cook for another 8 to 10 minutes or until tenderloin reaches 145°F (65°C). Remove pan from oven, cover, and let sit for 5 minutes before slicing.

5 In a food processor, combine 1 tablespoon olive oil, garlic, 1 tablespoon red wine vinegar, 1 tablespoon water, and ⅓ of the roasted carrots. Process until smooth.

6 In a large bowl, toss arugula with remaining 1 tablespoon red wine vinegar.

7 Arrange remaining carrots and arugula on a serving platter. Top with sliced pork tenderloin and drizzle with carrot romesco sauce.

Storage: Tenderloin is best served immediately, but can be refrigerated for up to 4 days.

NUTRITION

| Calories 317 | Saturated Fat 4g | Cholesterol 75mg | Carbohydrate 17g | Sugar 8g |
| Total Fat 17g | Unsaturated Fat 12g | Sodium 249mg | Dietary Fiber 5g | Protein 25g |

These beef and bacon meatloaf muffins are **packed with plenty of nutritious veggies** and topped with a creamy sweet potato purée.

Homestyle **Meatloaf Muffins**

 YIELD: **12 MUFFINS**   SERVING SIZE: **2 MUFFINS**   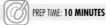 PREP TIME: **10 MINUTES**   COOK TIME: **20 MINUTES**

INGREDIENTS

2 TB. olive oil

2 cups yellow onion, chopped

2 celery stalks, chopped

2 carrots, peeled and chopped

4 cloves garlic, minced

1 tsp. marjoram

1 tsp. dried basil

1 tsp. dried oregano

¾ tsp. sea salt

1 lb. (450g) ground beef

2 TB. coconut flour

2 tsp. **Worcestershire Sauce**

¼ cup parsley, chopped

3 slices raw bacon, thinly sliced

3 cups sweet potato, peeled and chopped

2 TB. light coconut milk

1 TB. ghee

SPECIAL TOOLS

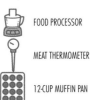

FOOD PROCESSOR

MEAT THERMOMETER

12-CUP MUFFIN PAN

METHOD

1 Preheat oven to 375°F (190°C). Heat olive oil in a large skillet over medium-high heat. Add onion, celery, carrots, and 3 teaspoons minced garlic. Cook for 5 minutes.

2 Add marjoram, basil, oregano, and ½ teaspoon sea salt. Cook for another 2 minutes.

3 Transfer vegetables to a large bowl. Add beef, coconut flour, Worcestershire Sauce, and parsley. Mix to combine.

4 Distribute meat mixture among 12 cups of a muffin pan. Press meat into muffin tin and top with 2 to 3 pieces of sliced bacon.

5 Bake meatloaf muffins for 20 minutes or until internal temperature reaches 155°F (68°C).

6 To make sweet potato purée, cover chopped sweet potatoes with water in a small saucepan. Bring to a boil. Reduce heat, cover, and simmer for 10 minutes or until fork-tender. Drain sweet potoatoes.

7 In a food processor, combine sweet potatoes, coconut milk, 1 clove garlic, remaining ¼ teaspoon sea salt, and ghee. Process for 30 seconds or until smooth.

8 Top meatloaf muffins with sweet potato purée before serving.

Storage: Meatloaf muffins can be refrigerated for up to one week or frozen for up to 3 months.

Serving Suggestion: Top meatloaf muffins with sweet potato topping and garnish with chopped cooked bacon and fresh chives. Serve with Triple-Berry Barbecue Sauce if desired.

NUTRITION

Calories 329

Total Fat 21g

Saturated Fat 8g

Unsaturated Fat 5g

Cholesterol 58mg

Sodium 517mg

Carbohydrate 20g

Dietary Fiber 5g

Sugar 5g

Protein 17g

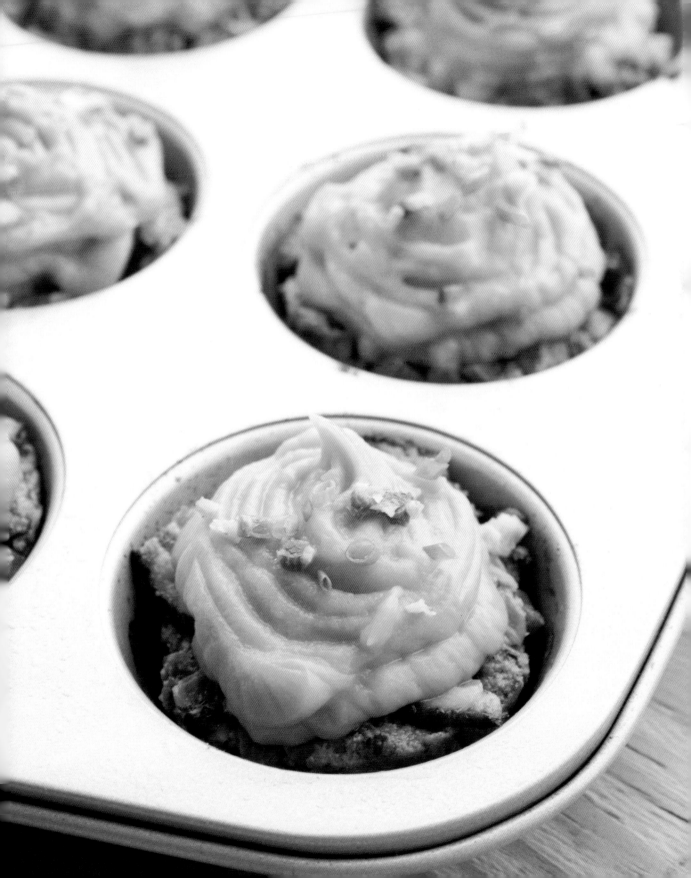

This blackened chicken has an enormous amount of flavor and **the perfect amount of char.** Use to top salads or mix into soups and stews.

Blackened Chicken Breast

 YIELD: **4 (3-OZ.; 75G) PIECES**   SERVING SIZE: **1 PIECE**   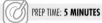 PREP TIME: **5 MINUTES**   COOK TIME: **6–10 MINUTES**

INGREDIENTS

1 lb. (450g) boneless, skinless chicken breast

1½ tsp. dried oregano

1½ tsp. dried thyme

1½ tsp. garlic powder

1 tsp. coconut sugar

½ tsp. **Seed-Free Curry Powder**

¼ tsp. sea salt

1 TB. olive oil

METHOD

1 Rinse chicken breasts under cold water and place in a large zipper-lock plastic bag. Using a meat tenderizer, pound meat into large, thin pieces.

2 On a large plate, combine oregano, thyme, garlic powder, coconut sugar, Seed-Free Curry Powder, and sea salt. Toss to mix.

3 Coat chicken breasts with spice mixture on both sides.

4 In a large skillet or grill pan, heat olive oil over high heat.

5 Cook seasoned chicken in olive oil for 3 to 5 minutes on each side until chicken is blackened slightly on the outside and cooked through.

6 Remove chicken from pan and let sit for 5 minutes until cutting or serving.

Storage: Refrigerate chicken for up to 3 days or freeze for up to 3 months.

Serving Suggestion: Use for Grilled Chicken Cobb Salad or Caribbean Chicken Salad, or serve over a bed of fresh spinach with chopped strawberries and Creamy Balsamic Dressing.

NUTRITION

Calories 164

Total Fat 4g

Saturated Fat 0g

Unsaturated Fat 3g

Cholesterol 10mg

Sodium 179mg

Carbohydrate 3g

Dietary Fiber 1g

Sugar 1g

Protein 26g

Coated in **apricot preserves and shredded coconut,** these sweet chicken fingers are crispy on the outside and tender on the inside.

Crispy **Chicken Strips** with **Mango Honey Sauce**

 YIELD: **8 STRIPS**   SERVING SIZE: **2 STRIPS**   PREP TIME: **15 MINUTES**   COOK TIME: **25 MINUTES**

INGREDIENTS

- 1 lb. (450g) boneless, skinless chicken breast
- 2 TB. coconut flour
- 2 TB. arrowroot powder
- ½ tsp. garlic powder
- ½ tsp. onion powder
- ¼ tsp. sea salt
- ½ cup light coconut milk
- ¼ cup apricot preserves
- 1 cup unsweetened shredded coconut
- ½ tsp. **Seed-Free Curry Powder**
- 1 cup mango, peeled and chopped
- 1 green onion, chopped
- 1 clove garlic, peeled
- 1 TB. honey
- 1 TB. apple cider vinegar
- 1 TB. lime juice

SPECIAL TOOLS

 FOOD PROCESSOR

METHOD

1 Preheat oven to 400°F (200°C). Line a baking sheet with foil.

2 Rinse chicken breasts under cold water and place in large zipper-lock plastic bag. Using a meat tenderizer, pound meat into large thin pieces. Remove chicken from bag and cut into 8 thin strips.

3 On a large plate, combine coconut flour, arrowroot powder, garlic powder, onion powder, and ⅛ tsp. sea salt.

4 In a small bowl, whisk together coconut milk and apricot preserves.

5 On a separate large plate, combine shredded coconut and Seed-Free Curry Powder.

6 Dredge each chicken strip in coconut flour mixture, dip in coconut milk mixture, and coat with the shredded coconut mixture. Place coated chicken strips on prepared baking sheet.

7 Bake for 15 minutes. Flip chicken strips and bake for another 15 minutes on the other side.

8 To make dipping sauce, combine mango, green onion, garlic, honey, apple cider vinegar, lime juice, and remaining ⅛ tsp. sea salt in a food processor. Process until smooth.

Storage: Crispy Chicken Strips are best enjoyed immediately.

Serving Suggestion: Serve with a side of Rosemary Sweet Potato Chips or Sea Salt Kale Crisps. Chicken strips can also be cut up and tossed on a salad.

NUTRITION

Calories 376
Total Fat 11g
Saturated Fat 8g
Unsaturated Fat 0g
Cholesterol 10mg
Sodium 91mg
Carbohydrate 39g
Dietary Fiber 9g
Sugar 22g
Protein 30g

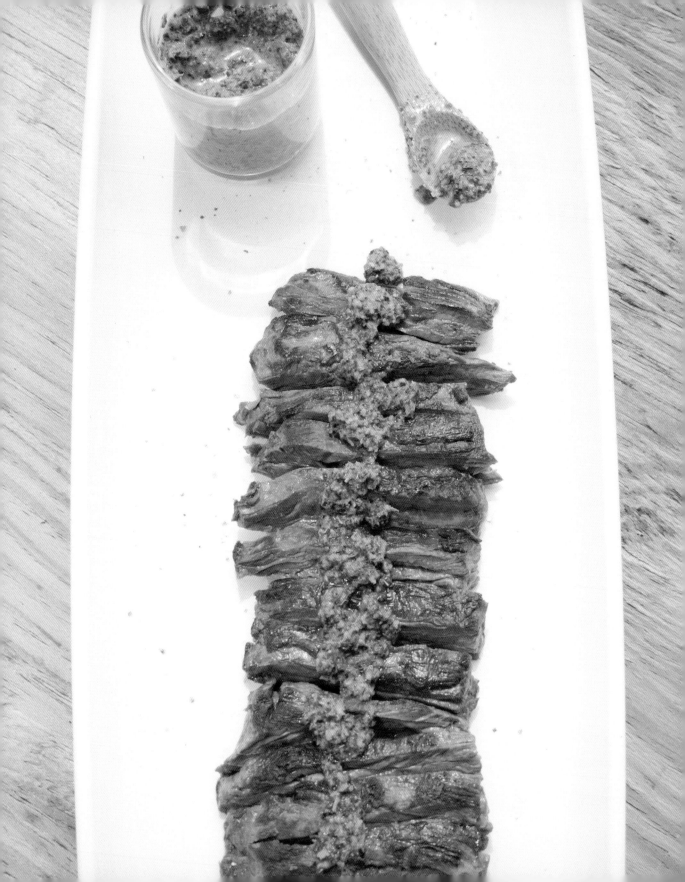

In Argentina, chimichurri sauce is served on grilled meats to add a burst of flavor. This **zesty, tangy sauce** is made with fresh herbs, garlic, and vinegar.

Chimichurri Skirt Steak

 YIELD: **4 (3-OZ.; 75G) PIECES**   SERVING SIZE: **1 PIECE**   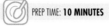 PREP TIME: **10 MINUTES**   COOK TIME: **5 MINUTES**

INGREDIENTS

1 lb. (450g) skirt steak

2 cups parsley, loosely packed

1 tsp. sea salt

2 TB. dried oregano

3 TB. lemon juice

3 TB. olive oil

3 TB. sherry vinegar

5 cloves garlic, peeled

½ shallot, peeled

SPECIAL TOOLS

 FOOD PROCESSOR

METHOD

1 Remove steak from refrigerator and allow it to come to room temperature.

2 Meanwhile, in a food processor, combine parsley, sea salt, oregano, lemon juice, olive oil, sherry vinegar, garlic, and shallot. Process for 30 seconds or until chimichurri is well combined.

3 Heat skillet over medium-high heat. Rinse steak, pat dry, and spinkle with a pinch of salt on both sides.

4 Cook steak for 3 minutes of each side until seared and brown.

5 Remove steak from pan, cover with foil and let sit 5 minutes before cutting.

6 Cut steak into thin slices and top with chimichurri sauce.

Storage: Steak is best enjoyed immediately. Chimichurri can be made ahead of time and refrigerated for up to 3 days.

Serving Suggestion: Serve with a warm side dish such as Garlic Caper Roasted Cauliflower or Savory Baked Butternut Squash.

NUTRITION

Calories 298

Total Fat 20g

Saturated Fat 5g

Unsaturated Fat 9g

Cholesterol 65mg

Sodium 675mg

Carbohydrate 6g

Dietary Fiber 2g

Sugar 1g

Protein 25g

An **overnight marinade of red wine and beef broth** infuses these lamb kabobs with savory, succulent flavor.

Burgundy **Lamb Kabobs**

 YIELD: **4 KABOBS**   SERVING SIZE: **1 KABOB**   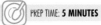 PREP TIME: **5 MINUTES**   COOK TIME: **6 TO 10 MINUTES**

INGREDIENTS

1 lb. (450g) lamb stew meat

2 cloves garlic, minced

1½ TB. dried parsley

2 tsp. olive oil

1 cup red wine

1 cup beef broth

¼ tsp. sea salt

½ tsp. lemon zest

1 large red onion

SPECIAL TOOLS

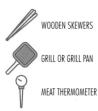

WOODEN SKEWERS

GRILL OR GRILL PAN

MEAT THERMOMETER

METHOD

1 In a large zipper-lock bag, combine lamb stew meat, garlic, parsley, olive oil, red wine, beef broth, sea salt, and lemon zest. Marinate 8 to 10 hours or overnight.

2 Place 4 wooden skewers in a shallow pan of water to soak for 30 minutes. Preheat grill or grill pan over high heat.

3 Cut onion into large pieces. Remove skewers from soaking water.

4 Assemble kabobs by threading marinated lamb stew meat and onions alternately onto each skewer. Reserve the excess meat marinade.

5 Cook the skewers on the grill for 6 to 10 minutes, turning occasionally, and brushing with reserved marinade as needed. Cook lamb until meat reaches 155°F (68°C).

Storage: Store leftover kabobs in the refrigerator for up to 4 days.

Serving Suggestion: Serve Burgundy Lamb Kabobs over a bed of lettuce and top with Greek Red Wine Vinaigrette for a quick and easy Greek salad.

Cooking these kabobs over high heat allows for most of the alcohol in the wine of the marinade to cook off before consuming.

NUTRITION

Calories **225**

Total Fat **8g**

Saturated Fat **3g**

Unsaturated Fat **2g**

Cholesterol **74mg**

Sodium **225mg**

Carbohydrate **3g**

Dietary Fiber **0g**

Sugar **1g**

Protein **24g**

This recipe takes ribs from the grill to the slow cooker, with **sweet and smoky barbecue flavor** you can enjoy year-round.

Triple-Berry **Barbecue Ribs**

 YIELD: **24 RIBS**   SERVING SIZE: **3 RIBS**   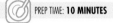 PREP TIME: **10 MINUTES**   COOK TIME: **7 HOURS**

INGREDIENTS

1½ racks of ribs (about 3 lb. [1.5kg] total)

½ tsp. sea salt

1 cup **Triple-Berry Barbecue Sauce**

SPECIAL TOOLS

 SLOW COOKER

METHOD

1 Cut each rack of ribs into smaller portions and season both sides with salt.

2 Brush ribs liberally with barbecue sauce and place in slow cooker, stacking them like shingles, one on top of the other.

3 Cook on high for 7 hours. Meat should be tender and falling off the bones.

Storage: Store leftover ribs in the refrigerator for up to 4 days.

Serving Suggestion: Serve ribs with additional barbecue sauce and a side of Honey Vinegar Tri-Colored Coleslaw.

NUTRITION

Calories 465	Saturated Fat 11g	Cholesterol 118g	Carbohydrate 11g	Sugar 8g
Total Fat 33g	Unsaturated Fat 19g	Sodium 801mg	Dietary Fiber 1g	Protein 30g

This salmon dinner is coated in a **simple homemade teriyaki sauce** made with all AIP-friendly ingredients.

Pineapple **Teriyaki Salmon**

 YIELD: **4 (3-OZ.; 75G) PIECES** SERVING SIZE: **1 PIECE** PREP TIME: **5 MINUTES** COOK TIME: **20 MINUTES**

INGREDIENTS

1 TB. coconut oil

2 cloves garlic, minced

½ cup coconut aminos

1 TB. honey

½ tsp. fish sauce

1 tsp. arrowroot powder

2 cups pineapple, chopped

1 lb. (450g) salmon, bones removed and skin on

METHOD

1 Preheat oven to 350°F (180°C).

2 In a small saucepan over medium-high heat, combine coconut oil and garlic. Stir to combine and cook for 2 minutes or until fragrant.

3 Reduce heat to medium-low and add coconut aminos, honey, and fish sauce.

4 Gradually whisk in arrowroot powder until sauce thickens. Remove from heat, cover, and set aside.

5 Line a baking dish with foil. Place pineapple at the bottom of the pan. Place salmon on top of pineapple and spoon sauce over the fish.

6 Bake for 15 minutes or until fish is flaky and pineapple is soft and caramelized.

Storage: Salmon is best served immediately, but leftovers can be refrigerated and used for lunch or dinner the following day.

Serving Suggestion: Serve salmon and grilled pineapple over Cauliflower Fried Rice.

Optional

Remove pineapple from the baking dish and transfer to a large skillet or grill over high heat. Cook for 5 to 10 minutes or until pineapple begins to char.

NUTRITION

Calories 221

Total Fat 8g

Saturated Fat 4g

Unsaturated Fat 26mg

Cholesterol 26mg

Sodium 1,002mg

Carbohydrate 15g

Dietary Fiber 1g

Sugar 11g

Protein 21g

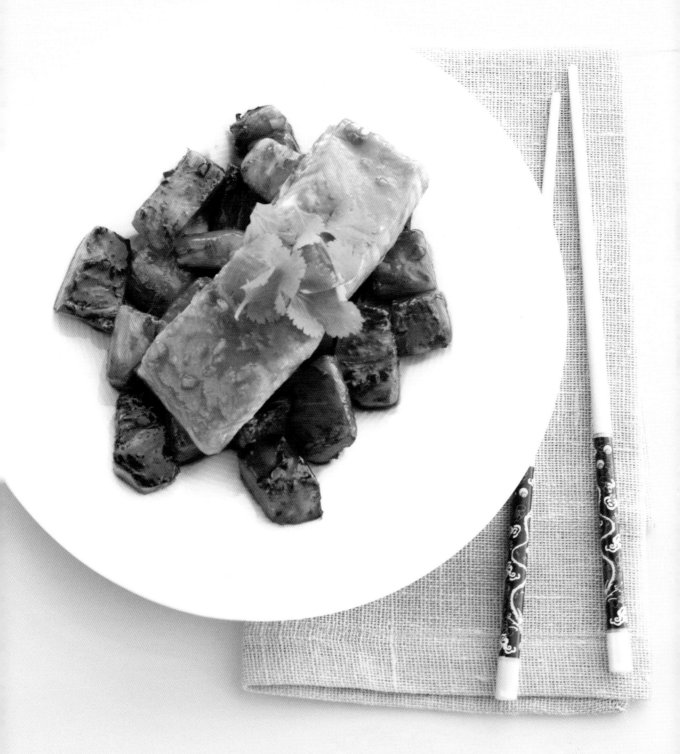

The **mild, sweet flavor and noodle-like texture** of spaghetti squash makes it an ideal substitute for traditional pasta noodles.

Herbed Baked
Spaghetti Squash

 YIELD: **5 CUPS**   SERVING SIZE: **1¼ CUP**   PREP TIME: **5 MINUTES**   COOK TIME: **45 MINUTES**

INGREDIENTS

1 medium spaghetti squash (about 4 lbs. [2kg])

2 TB. olive oil

1 TB. fresh rosemary, chopped

1 TB. fresh thyme, chopped

⅛ tsp. sea salt

METHOD

1 Preheat oven to 400°F (200°C). Line a baking sheet with foil.

2 Cut spaghetti squash lengthwise. Scoop out and discard seeds.

3 Place squash halves on baking sheet, flesh side up. Drizzle each half with olive oil, massaging the oil into the flesh to ensure it is well coated.

4 Sprinkle rosemary, thyme, and sea salt over the squash halves.

5 Bake for 30 to 45 minutes or until squash is fork tender.

6 Remove squash from oven and let cool for 10 to 20 minutes. Using a fork, carefully scrape the squash out of the skin.

Storage: Spaghetti squash can be stored in the refrigerator for up to 4 day.

Serving Suggestion: Serve spaghetti squash with Tomato-Less Pasta Sauce or Pork and Fennel Meatballs.

NUTRITION

Calories **100**

Total Fat **8g**

Saturated Fat **1g**

Unsaturated Fat **6g**

Cholesterol **0mg**

Sodium **80mg**

Carbohydrate **9g**

Dietary Fiber **2g**

Sugar **4g**

Protein **1g**

This nontraditional pasta dish features **crunchy, spiralized zucchini "noodles"** coated in a creamy pesto sauce made with garlic and basil.

Garlic Pesto
Zucchini Pasta

 YIELD: **16 CUPS**   SERVING SIZE: **2 CUPS**   PREP TIME: **10 MINUTES**   COOK TIME: **3 MINUTES**

INGREDIENTS

1 TB. plus ¾ cup olive oil

8 medium zucchini, spiralized

2 cups fresh basil

1 avocado, pit and skin removed

3 TB. lemon juice

3 cloves garlic, peeled

⅛ tsp. dried oregano

⅛ tsp. dried thyme

Dash sea salt

SPECIAL TOOLS

 SPIRALIZER

 FOOD PROCESSOR

METHOD

1 In a large skillet, heat 1 tablespoon olive oil over medium-high heat until hot. Add zucchini noodles and toss for 2 to 3 minutes until slightly tender. Remove from pan and set aside.

2 In a food processor, combine basil, avocado, lemon juice, remaining ¾ cup olive oil, garlic, oregano, thyme, and sea salt. Process for 30 seconds or until smooth.

3 In a large bowl, toss zucchini noodles with avocado pesto.

Storage: Zucchini pasta is best enjoyed immediately. Pesto can be stored in an airtight container in the refrigerator for up to 3 days.

A spiralizer tool turns vegetables into faux noodles. Whether you're making zucchini noodles, potato spirals, or rutabaga pasta, a spiralizer is an inexpensive way to create versatile, AIP-friendly noodles.

NUTRITION

Calories 237	Saturated Fat 3g	Cholesterol 0mg	Carbohydrate 5g	Sugar 3g
Total Fat 25g	Unsaturated Fat 18g	Sodium 18mg	Dietary Fiber 2g	Protein 2g

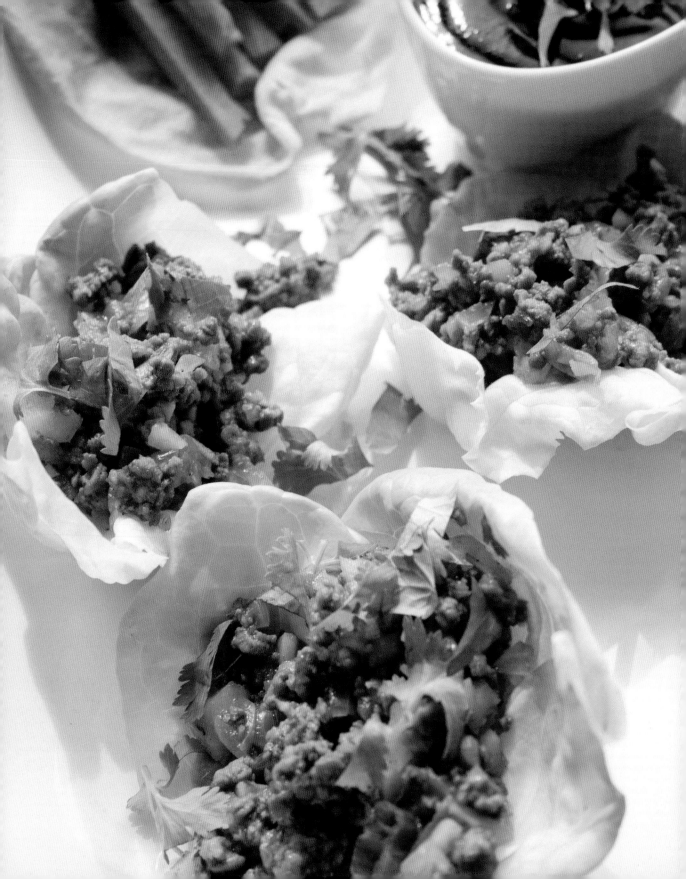

Dried plums, vinegar, and coconut aminos create a **tangy, sweet-and-salty plum sauce** perfect for dipping or drizzling over these healthy lettuce wraps.

Asian Turkey **Lettuce Wraps**

 YIELD: **16 WRAPS**   SERVING SIZE: **4 WRAPS**   PREP TIME: **10 MINUTES**   COOK TIME: **30 MINUTES**

INGREDIENTS

¼ cup pitted prunes (about 10 prunes)

2 TB. red onion, diced

3 TB. coconut aminos

1 TB. honey

1½ tsp. apple cider vinegar

3 tsp. minced garlic (about 3 cloves garlic)

⅛ tsp. sea salt

1 cup water

1 lb. (450g) ground turkey (preferably dark meat)

2 cups yellow onion, chopped (about 1 large onion)

1 TB. fresh ginger, peeled and minced

½ (8-oz.; 226g) can water chestnuts, drained and chopped

½ cup green onions, chopped

16 large butter lettuce leaves (about 2 heads lettuce)

METHOD

1 In a small saucepan over medium-high heat, combine prunes, red onion, 1 tablespoon coconut aminos, honey, apple cider vinegar, 1 teaspoon minced garlic, salt, and water.

2 Bring contents to a boil, cover, and reduce heat to low. Simmer for 20 minutes.

3 Remove sauce from the heat and transfer to blender. Blend until smooth and set aside.

4 In a large skillet over medium-high heat, combine ground turkey, yellow onion, remaining minced garlic, and ginger. Cook for 5 to 10 minutes or until meat is browned and onions are translucent and soft.

5 Add ¼ cup plum sauce and remaining 2 tablespoons coconut aminos to turkey mixture. Cook for another 5 minutes.

6 Remove pan from heat and stir in water chestnuts and green onions.

7 Spoon 2 tablespoons turkey mixture into each lettuce leaf. Drizzle with remaining plum sauce.

Storage: Lettuce wraps are best enjoyed immediately, but the turkey mixture can be refrigerated for up to 4 days.

Serving Suggestion: Top lettuce wraps with chopped cucumber, shredded carrots, and fresh cilantro if desired.

NUTRITION

Calories 333

Total Fat 14g

Saturated Fat 4g

Unsaturated Fat 0g

Cholesterol 85mg

Sodium 398mg

Carbohydrate 32g

Dietary Fiber 4g

Sugar 15g

Protein 20g

SPECIAL TOOLS

 BLENDER

Roasting this **delicate white fish with lemon and herbs** is a quick and easy way to bring out its mild, subtle flavor.

Lemon-Stuffed **Sea Bass**

 YIELD: **2 FISH**   SERVING SIZE: **1 FISH**   PREP TIME: **10 MINUTES**   COOK TIME: **20 MINUTES**

INGREDIENTS

2 whole sea bass, cleaned with gills and fins removed (about 2 lb.; 1kg)

2 TB. olive oil

2 cloves garlic, thinly sliced

1 lemon, sliced

4 sprigs rosemary

4 sprigs thyme

4 sprigs parsley

½ cup dry white wine

⅛ tsp. sea salt

METHOD

1 Preheat oven to 500°F (240°C).

2 Rub fish with 1 tablespoon olive oil on all sides.

3 Stuff each fish cavity with half of the garlic slices, 3 lemon slices, and 2 sprigs each of rosemary, thyme, and parsley.

4 Drizzle remaining 1 tablespoon olive oil into baking pan and place fish on top. Pour ¼ cup wine over the fish and sprinkle with sea salt.

5 Bake for 10 minutes. Flip fish, pour remaining ¼ cup white wine over fish, and bake for another 10 minutes.

6 Remove from oven and squeeze remaining lemon slices over fish before serving.

Storage: Sea bass is best served immediately.

NUTRITION

Calories 456	Saturated Fat 2g	Cholesterol 29mg	Carbohydrate 5g	Sugar 1g
Total Fat 16g	Unsaturated Fat 11g	Sodium 177mg	Dietary Fiber 1g	Protein 54g

A zesty coconut milk sauce unites the flavors of tender, **sweet sea scallops and crispy, salty bacon** in this decadent dish.

Bacon-Wrapped **Scallops**

 YIELD: **12 SCALLOPS**   SERVING SIZE: **3 SCALLOPS**   PREP TIME: **10 MINUTES**   COOK TIME: **12 MINUTES**

INGREDIENTS

1 lb. (450g) large sea scallops

12 slices of bacon

¼ cup light coconut milk

Juice of 1 lime

2 TB. cilantro, chopped

METHOD

1 Preheat broiler. Line a baking dish with foil.

2 Rinse scallops under cold water and pat dry with a paper towel.

3 Roll each scallop in a slice of bacon and secure with a toothpick.

4 Place scallops in baking dish and broil for 6 minutes.

5 Flip scallops and broil for another 6 minutes until tops are golden brown and scallops are cooked through.

6 In a small bowl, whisk together coconut milk, lime juice, and cilantro.

7 Drizzle cooked scallops with coconut milk mixture before serving.

Storage: Scallops are best served immediately.

NUTRITION

Calories 300	Saturated Fat 6g	Cholesterol 72mg	Carbohydrate 7g	Sugar 2g
Total Fat 16g	Unsaturated Fat 0g	Sodium 1,169mg	Dietary Fiber 0g	Protein 32g

Indulge in the **rich, gamey flavor of duck** paired with **savory leeks, chewy figs,** and a **sticky honey glaze**.

Roast Duck with Shallots, Figs, and Honey

 YIELD: **4 CUPS**   SERVING SIZE: **½ CUP**   PREP TIME: **15 MINUTES**   COOK TIME: **1 HOUR**

INGREDIENTS

2 (½ lb.; 225g each) duck breasts, skin on

⅛ tsp. sea salt

3 tsp. fresh thyme, chopped

2 TB. olive oil

4 cups leeks, white and green parts, thinly sliced (2 large leeks)

2 cups carrots, peeled and chopped (4–5 carrots)

2 TB. honey

½ cup plus 1 tsp. red wine

2 oz. pancetta, chopped

1 cup dried figs, chopped and stems removed

½ cup vegetable broth

SPECIAL TOOLS

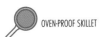 OVEN-PROOF SKILLET

METHOD

1 Preheat oven to 350°F (180°C). Rinse duck breasts under cold water and pat dry. With a sharp knife, score the fat of the duck breast in a crisscross pattern. Season duck breasts with salt and 2 teaspoons thyme.

2 In a large skillet, heat olive oil over medium-high heat. Add leeks and carrots. Cook for 20 minutes or until vegetables are soft.

3 Push vegetables to the side and place duck breasts, skin side down, in the center of the pan. Cook, undisturbed, for 10 minutes.

5 In a small bowl, whisk together honey and 1 teaspoon red wine. Flip duck breasts and brush with honey mixture.

6 Transfer skillet to the oven and roast for 10 minutes. Brush duck breasts with remaining honey mixture and roast for another 10 minutes or until internal temperature reaches 165°F (74°C).

7 In a saucepan over medium-high heat, cook pancetta for 3 minutes or until crispy. Add figs, remaining ½ cup red wine, vegetable broth, and remaining 1 teaspoon thyme. Bring contents to a boil, reduce heat, and simmer for 10 minutes.

8 Remove skillet from oven and let sit for 5 minutes. Top with fig sauce before serving.

Storage: Duck is best served immediately.

NUTRITION

Calories 577	Saturated Fat 6g	Cholesterol 10mg	Carbohydrate 53g	Sugar 33g
Total Fat 25g	Unsaturated Fat 14g	Sodium 356mg	Dietary Fiber 7g	Protein 37g

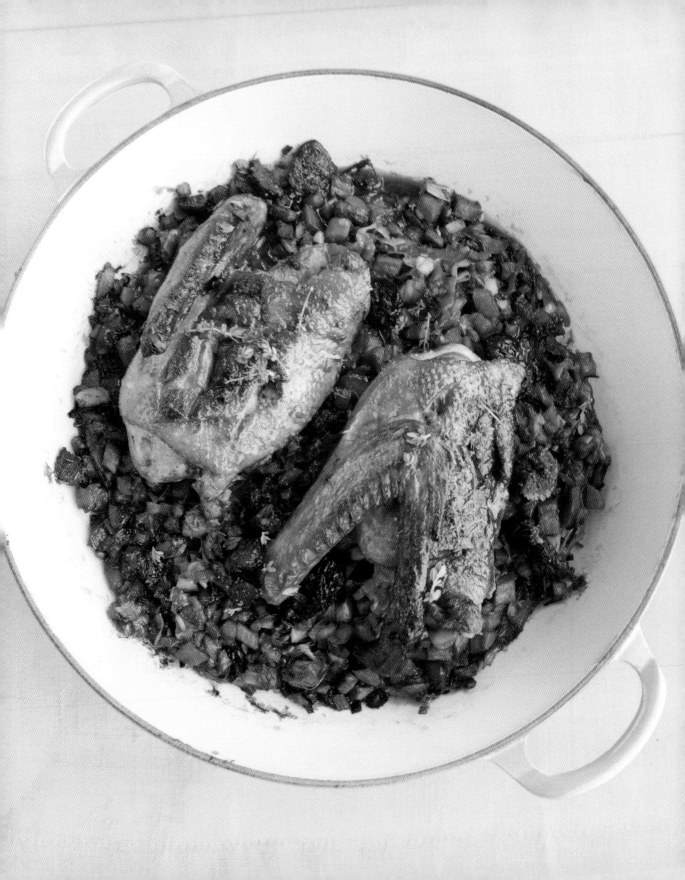

Fennel, fresh herbs, and lemon zest bring **bright, spring-like flavors** to these easy and versatile meatballs.

Pork and Fennel **Meatballs**

 YIELD: **48 MEATBALLS**   SERVING SIZE: **6 MEATBALLS**   PREP TIME: **1 HOUR**   COOK TIME: **15 MINUTES**

INGREDIENTS

¾ cup yellow onion, chopped (½ medium onion)

½ cup fennel, chopped (½ fennel bulb)

1 clove garlic

¼ cup puncetta, chopped

¼ cup parsley

1 TB. fresh rosemary

1 TB. fresh oregano

1 lb. ground pork

1 TB. lemon juice

1 tsp. lemon zest

1 TB. arrowroot powder

Dash sea salt

1 TB. olive oil

SPECIAL TOOLS

 FOOD PROCESSOR

 MEAT THERMOMETER

METHOD

1 Combine onion, fennel, garlic, pancetta, parsley, rosemary, and oregano in a food processor. Pulse until finely chopped.

2 Transfer herb mixture to a large bowl. Add ground pork, lemon juice, lemon zest, arrowroot powder, and salt. Mix until well combined.

3 With clean hands, form 1-tablespoon portions of meat mixture into balls (you should have about 48 meatballs).

4 In a large, deep skillet, heat olive oil over medium-high heat. Add meatballs and cook for 8 to 10 minutes, turning frequently until browned on all sides and internal temperature reaches at least 160°F (70°C).

5 Using a slotted spoon, remove meatballs from pan and set aside on a plate lined with a clean paper towel to soak up any remaining grease. Allow to cool slightly before serving.

Storage: Refrigerate for 5 days or freeze for up to 3 months.

Serving Suggestion: Serve with Herbed Baked Spaghetti Squash and Tomato-Less Pasta Sauce or in Wild Mushroom Meatball Stew.

NUTRITION

Calories 249

Total Fat 20g

Saturated Fat 7g

Unsaturated Fat 11g

Cholesterol 58mg

Sodium 142mg

Carbohydrate 4g

Dietary Fiber 1g

Sugar 0g

Protein 14g

These burgers feature lean bison and are spiced with the robust **Mediterranean** flavors of garlic and curry.

Middle Eastern **Bison Burgers**

 YIELD: **4 PATTIES**   SERVING SIZE: **1 PATTY**   PREP TIME: **10 MINUTES**   COOK TIME: **10 MINUTES**

INGREDIENTS

- 1 lb. (450g) ground bison
- ½ cup red onion, chopped (¼ large onion)
- ¼ cup parsley, chopped
- 2 cloves garlic, minced
- 2 tsp. **Seed-Free Curry Powder**
- 1 tsp. salt
- 1 TB. olive oil

METHOD

1 In a large bowl, combine ground bison, red onion, parsley, garlic, Seed-Free Curry Powder, and salt.

2 With clean hands, mix ingredients until well combined and form into 4 tightly packed hamburger patties.

3 In a large skillet, heat olive oil over medium-high heat. Add burger patties and cook, undisturbed, for 4 minutes.

4 Flip burgers and cook for another 4 minutes on the other side.

Storage: Refrigerate for 5 days or freeze for up to 3 months.

Serving Suggestion: Serve over a bed of lettuce topped with Fool-Proof Caramelized Onions and a side of Rosemary Sweet Potato Chips.

NUTRITION

Calories 291	Saturated Fat 8g	Cholesterol 79mg	Carbohydrate 2g	Sugar 0g
Total Fat 22g	Unsaturated Fat 11g	Sodium 660mg	Dietary Fiber 0g	Protein 22g

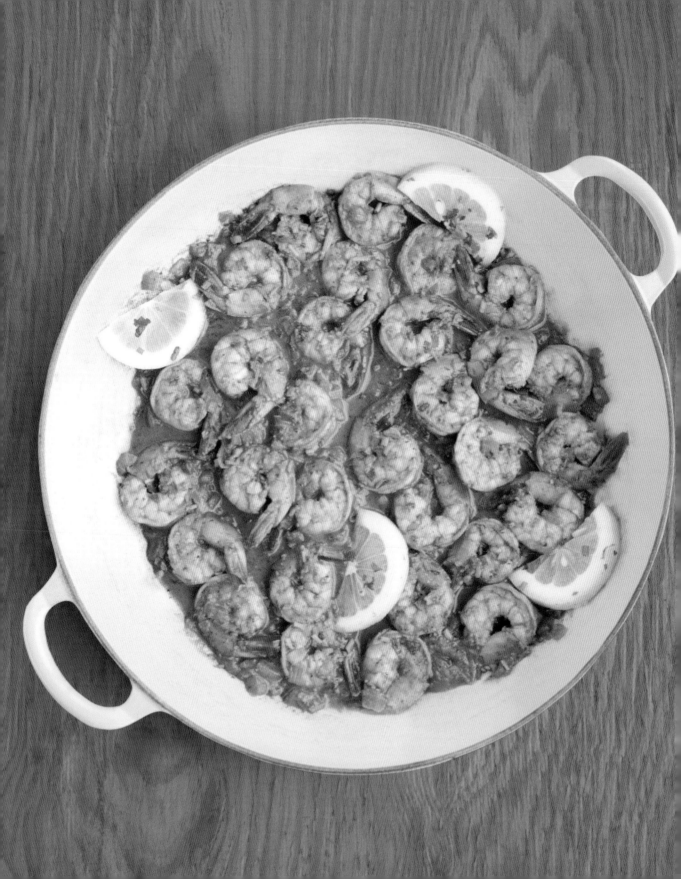

These shrimp are sautéed New Orleans style in a **lemon butter sauce spiked with Worcestershire Sauce** and white wine.

New Orleans
Barbecue Shrimp

 YIELD: **30 SHRIMP**   SERVING SIZE: **10 SHRIMP**   PREP TIME: **10 MINUTES**   COOK TIME: **20 MINUTES**

INGREDIENTS

1 lb. (450g) shrimp, peeled and deveined

1½ tsp. **Seed-Free Curry Powder**

1 TB. ghee

1 TB. olive oil

1 cup yellow onion, chopped (about ½ large onion)

2 cloves garlic, minced

¼ cup **Worcestershire Sauce**

⅓ cup dry white wine

1 cup vegetable broth

1 bay leaf

Juice of 1 lemon

1 TB. light coconut milk

METHOD

1 Rinse shrimp under cold water and pat dry with a paper towel.

2 In a large bowl, toss shrimp with Seed-Free Curry Powder until well coated.

3 In a skillet over medium heat, combine ghee, oil, onion, and garlic. Cook for 5 minutes or until onions become soft.

4 Add Worcestershire Sauce, white wine, vegetable broth, bay leaf, and lemon juice to the skillet. Bring contents to a boil.

5 Reduce heat to low and simmer, uncovered, for 10 minutes.

6 Stir in shrimp and cook for 5 minutes until pink and cooked through. Stir in coconut milk.

Storage: Shrimp are best served immediately, but can be refrigerated for up to 3 days.

Serving Suggestion: Serve over Parsnip Purée or Rutabaga Purée.

NUTRITION

Calories 325
Total Fat 12g
Saturated Fat 4g
Unsaturated Fat 6g
Cholesterol 12mg
Sodium 695mg
Carbohydrate 16g
Dietary Fiber 1g
Sugar 8g
Protein 34g

A **sweet and savory glaze** gives this baked salmon a delicious mouthful of flavor in every bite.

Maple Balsamic **Glazed Salmon**

 YIELD: **4 (3-OZ.; 75G) PIECES**   SERVING SIZE: **1 PIECE**   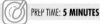 PREP TIME: **5 MINUTES**   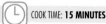 COOK TIME: **15 MINUTES**

INGREDIENTS

1 lb. (450g) salmon, skin on, cut into 4 pieces

¼ cup maple syrup

¼ cup balsamic vinegar

2 cloves garlic, minced

1 TB. olive oil

1 TB. molasses

⅛ tsp. sea salt

METHOD

1 Preheat oven to 425°F (220°C).

2 Line a baking sheet with foil. Place salmon on baking sheet, skin side down.

3 In a small bowl, whisk together maple syrup, balsamic vinegar, garlic, olive oil, molasses, and salt.

4 Brush salmon with glaze, reserving any excess. Bake 5 minutes, brush with more glaze, and return to oven. Repeat twice more, baking salmon for a total of 15 minutes.

5 Allow salmon to cool on pan for a few minutes before serving. Lift the flesh from the skin to serve (the skin will stick to the foil). Discard the skin and foil.

Storage: Salmon can be stored in the refrigerator for up to 3 days.

Serving Suggestion: Serve salmon atop a Classic Kale Salad or over mixed greens with Sweet Red Raspberry Vinaigrette.

NUTRITION

Calories 245	Saturated Fat 1g	Cholesterol 59mg	Carbohydrate 20g	Sugar 20g
Total Fat 7g	Unsaturated Fat 6g	Sodium 142mg	Dietary Fiber 0g	Protein 23g

Halibut is layered with zucchini, shallots, garlic, and lemon and **cooked** *en papillote*—in a parchment pouch.

Lemon Baked Halibut

 YIELD: **4 (3-OZ.; 75G) PIECES**   SERVING SIZE: **1 PIECE** 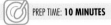 PREP TIME: **10 MINUTES**   COOK TIME: **20 MINUTES**

INGREDIENTS

2 lemons

2 small zucchini, sliced lengthwise

1 shallot, thinly sliced

1 lb. (450g) fresh halibut, skin on, cut into 4 pieces

2 cloves garlic, minced

2 TB. fresh thyme, chopped

⅛ tsp. sea salt

2 TB. ghee, melted

METHOD

1 Preheat oven to 400°F (200°F). Cut 4 17×12-inch (43×30cm) pieces of parchment paper.

2 Cut 1 lemon horizontally into 8 slices. Place 2 lemon slices on top of each piece of parchment paper. Top lemons with 2 slices of zucchini each.

3 Top zucchini with a few slices of shallots followed by a fish filet.

4 Top each fish fillet with garlic, thyme, and sea salt.

5 Fold parchment paper over the layered fish, folding and rolling the edges to create a tight pouch of paper with the fish inside.

6 Place parchment pouch on a baking sheet and bake for 20 minutes.

7 Squeeze juice from remaining lemon into a small bowl. Whisk in ghee and a pinch of salt.

8 Remove pan from oven and cut open the parchment paper to remove veggies and fish. Drizzle with lemon ghee before serving.

Storage: Halibut can be stored in the refrigerator for up to 3 days.

Serving Suggestion: Serve with a side of roasted or steamed vegetables.

NUTRITION

Calories **217**

Total Fat **10g**

Saturated Fat **5g**

Unsaturated Fat **3g**

Cholesterol **54mg**

Sodium **128mg**

Carbohydrate **9g**

Dietary Fiber **3g**

Sugar **3g**

Protein **26g**

In this recipe, **carrots, broccoli, and zucchini** take the place of traditional noodles, while tangy fish sauce and vinegar **mimic classic pad thai** flavor.

Pad Thai Noodles

 YIELD: **3 CUPS**   SERVING SIZE: **1 CUP**   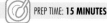 PREP TIME: **15 MINUTES**   COOK TIME: **10 MINUTES**

INGREDIENTS

4 medium carrots, peeled

1 medium zucchini, peeled

2 TB. coconut oil

3 cloves garlic, minced

¼ cup fish sauce

2 TB. coconut aminos

¼ cup lime juice

1 TB. apple cider vinegar

3 cups broccoli slaw

½ cup green onions, chopped

¼ cup fresh cilantro, chopped

1 lime, cut into wedges

METHOD

1 Using a vegetable peeler, create carrot and zucchini "noodles" by shaving the vegetables in long, thin strokes.

2 In a large skillet, combine coconut oil and garlic. Sauté for 2 minutes or until soft.

3 Add fish sauce, coconut aminos, lime juice, and apple cider vinegar. Simmer for 5 minutes or until sauce is reduced by half.

4 Add carrots, zucchini, broccoli slaw, and green onions. Toss to coat and cook for 2 to 3 minutes.

5 Remove pan from heat and top with cilantro and lime wedges.

Storage: Pad Thai Noodles are best served immediately.

Serving Suggestion: Top noodles with your choice of cooked chicken or shrimp.

Preshredded broccoli slaw can be found near the bagged lettuce at most supermarkets. Its sturdy, crunchy texture makes an excellent stand-in for noodles in stir-fries.

NUTRITION

Calories 199	Saturated Fat 9g	Cholesterol 0mg	Carbohydrate 17g	Sugar 8g
Total Fat 10g	Unsaturated Fat 0g	Sodium 2,301mg	Dietary Fiber 6g	Protein 11g

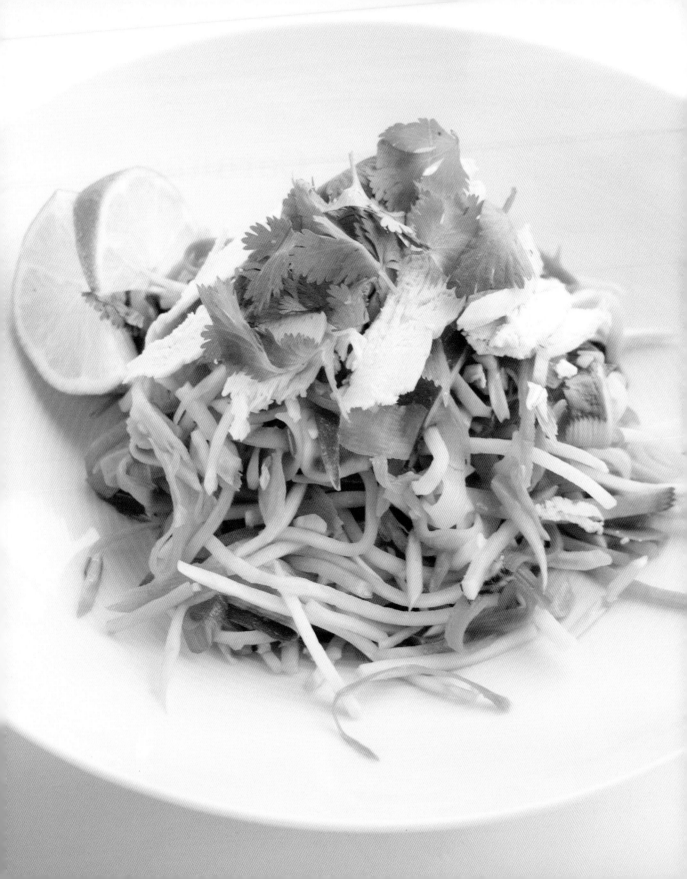

The simple ingredients of onion, garlic, and orange come together to create a **juicy pulled pork with a tangy citrus flavor.**

Orange Pulled Pork **Carnitas**

 YIELD: **5 CUPS**   SERVING SIZE: ¾ CUP   PREP TIME: **15 MINUTES**   COOK TIME: **8 HOURS**

INGREDIENTS

3½ lb. (1.6kg) boneless pork shoulder

2 TB. olive oil

¼ tsp. sea salt

1 TB. dried oregano

1½ tsp. **Seed-Free Curry Powder**

2 cups red onion, thinly sliced (1 large onion)

5 cloves garlic, sliced

1 orange, halved

SPECIAL TOOLS

 SLOW COOKER

METHOD

1 Rinse pork shoulder under cold water and pat dry with paper towels.

2 In a small bowl, combine olive oil, salt, oregano, and Seed-Free Curry Powder. Rub mixture on all sides of pork shoulder.

3 Place pork shoulder in slow cooker. Add onions and garlic to slow cooker, on top of the pork shoulder.

4 Squeeze the orange over the vegetables and meat and toss the remainder of the orange into the slow cooker. Cover and cook on low for 8 hours.

5 Remove meat from slow cooker and place on cutting board. Let meat cool slightly and pull it apart using two forks to shred it.

Storage: Refrigerate for 5 days or freeze for up to 3 months.

Serving Suggestion: Top carnitas with chopped cilantro, white onion, and avocado to add Mexican flair, or add Triple-Berry Barbecue Sauce for a smoky summer dish.

NUTRITION

Calories 514

Total Fat 39g

Saturated Fat 13g

Unsaturated Fat 22g

Cholesterol 141g

Sodium 203mg

Carbohydrate 4g

Dietary Fiber 1g

Sugar 2g

Protein 35g

A sweet potato chip coating gives these fish sticks a **crunchy outer texture** and the perfect balance of sweet and salty flavors.

Sweet Potato Chip **Fish Sticks**

 YIELD: **16 FISH STICKS**   SERVING SIZE: **2 FISH STICKS**   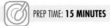 PREP TIME: **15 MINUTES**   COOK TIME: **15 MINUTES**

INGREDIENTS

6 cups **Rosemary Sweet Potato Chips**

2 tsp. dried oregano

¼ cup light coconut milk

1 TB. lemon juice

1 lb. (450g) cod, cut into 2-inch (5cm) pieces

SPECIAL TOOLS

 FOOD PROCESSOR

METHOD

1 Preheat oven to 425°F (220°C).

2 In a food processor, process Rosemary Sweet Potato Chips until finely chopped.

3 In a shallow dish, combine sweet potato chip crumbs and oregano.

4 In a small bowl, whisk together coconut milk and lemon juice.

5 Line baking sheet with foil. Place a wire rack on the baking sheet.

6 Dip each piece of fish into coconut mixture, coat with sweet potato mixture, and place on wire rack.

7 Bake for 15 minutes or until fish is flaky and cooked through.

Storage: Refrigerate for up to 2 days or freeze for up to 1 month.

Serving Suggestion: Serve with a side of Tartar Sauce Mayo.

NUTRITION

Calories **271**

Total Fat **17g**

Saturated Fat **3g**

Unsaturated Fat **13g**

Cholesterol **24mg**

Sodium **168mg**

Carbohydrate **18g**

Dietary Fiber **3g**

Sugar **6g**

Protein **12g**

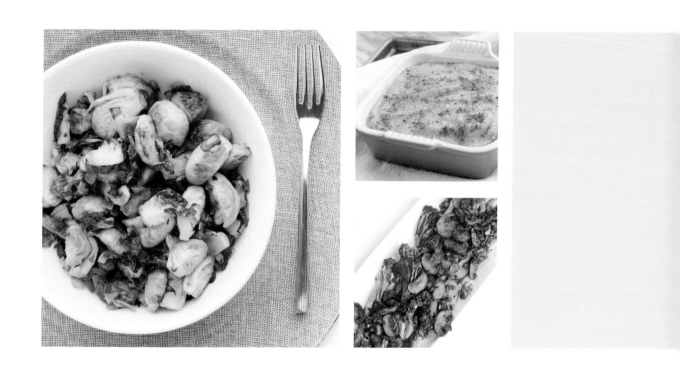

CHAPTER 6

Side Dishes

In this warm side dish, the **nuttiness of roasted cauliflower** is enhanced by the **zesty, briny flavors** of lemon and capers.

Garlic Caper
Roasted Cauliflower

 YIELD: **2 CUPS**   SERVING SIZE: **1 CUP**   PREP TIME: **10 MINUTES**   COOK TIME: **25 MINUTES**

INGREDIENTS

5 cups cauliflower florets
   (1 meduium head cauliflower)

1 TB. coconut oil, melted

2 TB. olive oil

¼ cup fresh parsley, chopped

1 TB. lemon zest

¼ cup lemon juice

2 TB. nonpareil capers, chopped

1 clove garlic, minced

METHOD

1 Preheat oven to 400°F (200°C). Line a baking sheet with foil.

2 Spread cauliflower on a baking sheet and drizzle with coconut oil, massaging it into the florets to ensure they are well coated.

3 Roast cauliflower for 15 minutes. Flip cauliflower pieces and roast for another 10 minutes or until edges are crisp and golden brown.

4 In a small bowl, combine olive oil, parsley, lemon zest, lemon juice, capers, and garlic. Whisk to combine.

5 In a large bowl, toss roasted cauliflower with dressing before serving.

Storage: Cauliflower is best enjoyed immediately, but can be refrigerated for up to 48 hours.

Serving Suggestion: Serve cauliflower as a savory side dish to Chimichurri Skirt Steak or Blackened Chicken Breast.

NUTRITION

Calories 269

Total Fat 21g

Saturated Fat 8g

Unsaturated Fat 12g

Cholesterol 0mg

Sodium 92mg

Carbohydrate 19g

Dietary Fiber 8g

Sugar 8g

Protein 6g

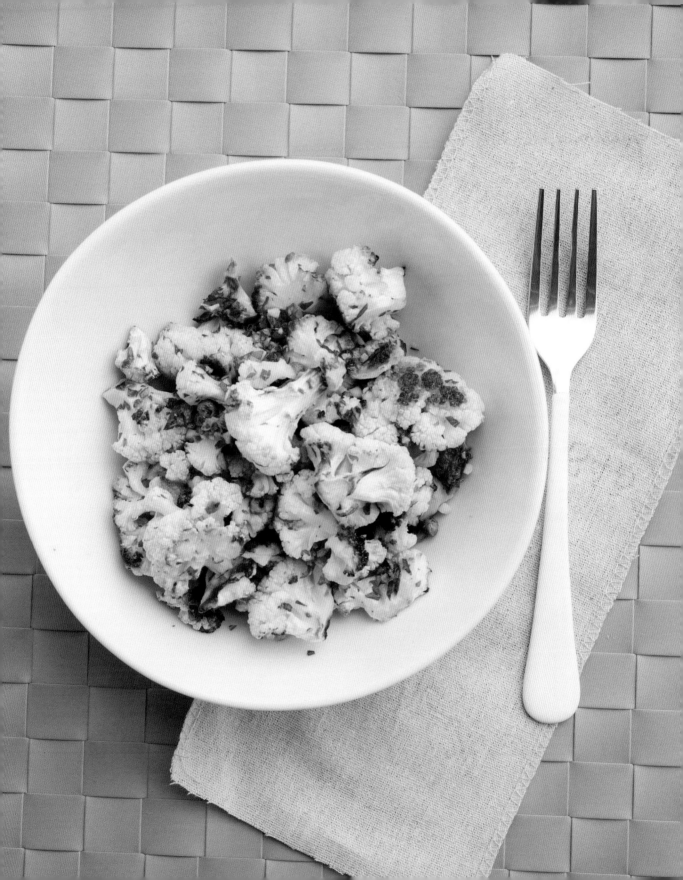

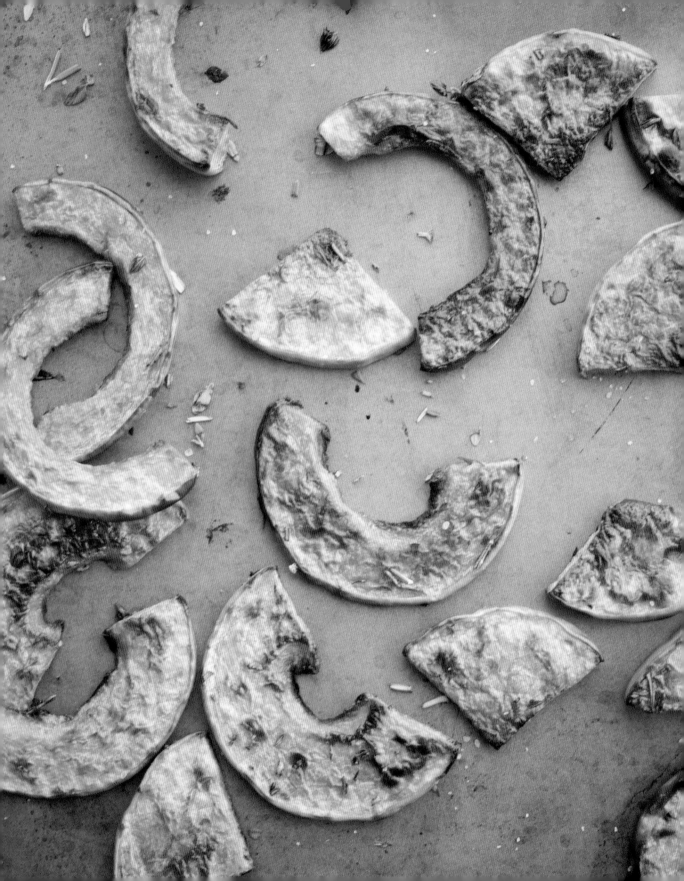

This quick and satisfying side dish features **butternut squash and savory fresh herbs** roasted until tender and golden brown.

Savory Baked
Butternut Squash

 YIELD: **4 CUPS**   SERVING SIZE: **1 CUP**   PREP TIME: **5 MINUTES**   COOK TIME: **20 MINUTES**

INGREDIENTS

1 butternut squash, sliced and seeds removed

1 TB. olive oil

½ tsp. fresh rosemary, chopped

½ tsp. fresh thyme, chopped

Pinch sea salt

METHOD

1 Preheat oven to 400°F (200°C). Line a baking sheet with foil.

2 Place squash on baking sheet and drizzle with olive oil, massaging it into the squash with clean hands to ensure it is well coated.

3 Sprinkle squash with rosemary, thyme, and sea salt.

4 Roast squash for 10 minutes. Flip and roast for another 10 minutes until squash is golden brown and fork-tender.

Storage: Squash can be refrigerated for up to 4 days.

Serving Suggestion: Serve squash as a savory side dish to Chimichurri Skirt Steak or Apple Cider Pork Chops.

Butternut squash is usually prepared by removing and discarding the thin, beige skin. However, the skin softens when roasted and is, in fact, edible.

NUTRITION

| Calories 93 | Saturated Fat 0g | Cholesterol 0mg | Carbohydrate 16g | Sugar 3g |
| Total Fat 4g | Unsaturated Fat 3g | Sodium 44mg | Dietary Fiber 3g | Protein 1g |

Roasting green beans in balsamic vinegar gives this **crunchy side dish** a **delicious tangy bite.**

Roasted Balsamic
Green Beans

 YIELD: **4 CUPS**   SERVING SIZE: **1 CUP**   PREP TIME: **5 MINUTE**   COOK TIME: **10 MINUTES**

INGREDIENTS

1 lb. (450g) green beans, ends trimmed and discarded

1 TB. olive oil

4 tsp. balsamic vinegar

Pinch sea salt

METHOD

1 Preheat oven to 400°F (200°C). Line a baking sheet with foil.

2 Place green beans on baking sheet. Drizzle with olive oil and 3 teaspoons balsamic vinegar.

3 Massage the oil and vinegar into the green beans with clean hands. Sprinkle with sea salt.

4 Roast green beans for 10 minutes or until tender.

5 Remove pan from oven and toss green beans with remaining 1 teaspoon balsamic vinegar before serving.

Storage: Green beans can be stored in the refrigerator for up to 3 days.

NUTRITION

Calories 60	Saturated Fat 0g	Cholesterol 0mg	Carbohydrate 6g	Sugar 3g
Total Fat 3g	Unsaturated Fat 2g	Sodium 31mg	Dietary Fiber 2g	Protein 1g

This cranberry relish is packed with nutrient-dense whole foods, including **tart cranberries, chewy golden raisins,** and **crunchy apples.**

Orange Cranberry **Relish**

 YIELD: **4 CUPS**   SERVING SIZE: **⅔ CUP**   PREP TIME: **5 MINUTES**   COOK TIME: **30 MINUTES**

INGREDIENTS

4 cups whole cranberries

¾ cup maple syrup

½ cup golden raisins

2 tsp. ground cinnamon

1 tsp. ground ginger

1 cup water

1 cup yellow onion, chopped (about ½ onion)

2 cups apple, peeled and chopped (about 1 medium apple)

1 cup orange juice

METHOD

1 In a medium saucepan, combine cranberries, maple syrup, raisins, cinnamon, ginger, and water.

2 Heat over medium-high heat, uncovered, for 15 minutes or until cranberries have popped and begin to soften.

3 Add onion, apple, and orange juice. Continue cooking, uncovered, for another 15 minutes until mixture has thickened.

Storage: Cranberry relish can be refrigerated for up to 1 week or frozen for up to 3 months.

NUTRITION

Calories 225	Saturated Fat 0g	Cholesterol 0mg	Carbohydrate 58g	Sugar 45g
Total Fat 0g	Unsaturated Fat 0g	Sodium 7mg	Dietary Fiber 6g	Protein 1g

Pan-searing brussels sprouts in **rich and flavorful** bacon fat renders them tender and delicious, with **crispy, caramelized outer leaves.**

Pan-Seared **Brussels Sprouts** with Bacon

 YIELD: **3 CUPS**   SERVING SIZE: ½ **CUP**   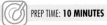 PREP TIME: **10 MINUTES**   COOK TIME: **25 MINUTES**

INGREDIENTS

4 slices bacon, chopped

1 lb. (450g) brussels sprouts, trimmed and quartered

1 cup yellow onion, chopped (about ½ onion)

METHOD

1 In a large skillet, cook bacon over medium-high heat for 5 minutes or until crispy.

2 Remove bacon from pan and place on a clean plate lined with a paper towel to absorb excess grease.

3 In remaining bacon fat, cook onion and brussels sprouts for 15 to 20 minutes or until tender and caramelized.

4 Remove pan from heat and stir bacon into brussels sprouts mixture.

Storage: These brussels sprouts are best served immediately, but can be stored in the refrigerator for up to 2 days.

Serving Suggestion: Serve as a side dish with Lemon Baked Halibut or Lemon-Stuffed Sea Bass.

NUTRITION

Calories 60	Saturated Fat 1g	Cholesterol 3mg	Carbohydrate 7g	Sugar 2g
Total Fat 3g	Unsaturated Fat 0g	Sodium 109mg	Dietary Fiber 3g	Protein 4g

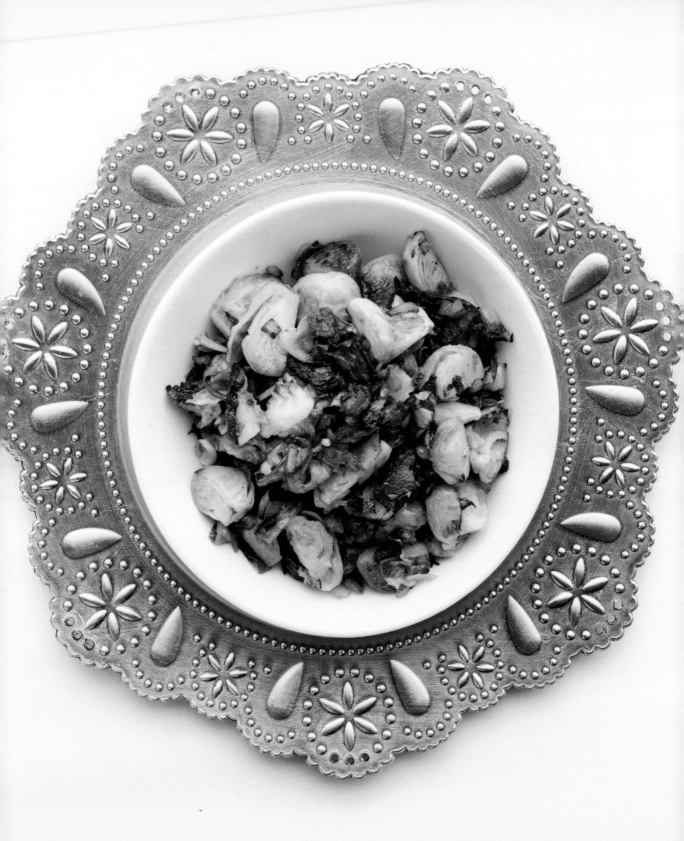

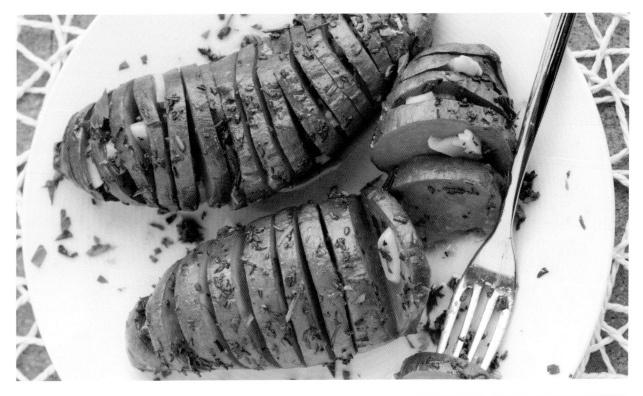

How to Hasselback

The potatoes in this dish are cut in a style called "Hasselback," named for the Swedish restaurant where the technique originated. The thin slices not only look impressive, but provide pockets for flavorful additions like garlic, butter, and fresh herbs. Although it appears complex, it's easy to prepare.

1 Using a sharp knife, slice a portion of the potato flesh from the base of the potato to create a flat, even surface for the potato to sit on.

2 Slice the potatoes the short way, creating cuts about ⅛-inch (3mm) apart, making sure not to cut entirely through the potato and stopping about ¼ inch (6mm) from the bottom.

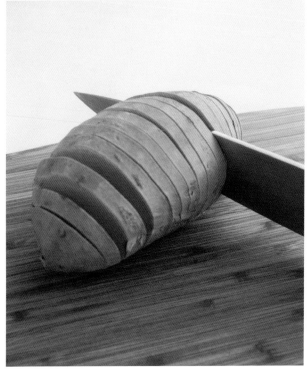

Swap traditional baked potatoes for these accordion-sliced sweet potatoes, which are **crisp on the outside** and **soft and tender on the inside**.

Hasselback **Sweet Potatoes**

 YIELD: **4 POTATOES**   SERVING SIZE: **1 POTATO**   PREP TIME: **10 MINUTES**   COOK TIME: **50 MINUTES**

INGREDIENTS

- 4 medium sweet potatoes
- 4 garlic cloves, thinly sliced
- 3 TB. ghee, melted
- 1 TB. fresh rosemary, finely chopped
- 1 TB. fresh sage, finely chopped
- ¼ tsp. salt

METHOD

1 Preheat oven to 375°F (190°C).

2 Hasselback the potatoes and press a piece of sliced garlic into each of the potato grooves.

3 Place potatoes in a baking dish. Brush with melted ghee and sprinkle with rosemary, sage, and salt. Cover pan with foil.

4 Bake for 50 minutes or until potatoes are fork-tender.

5 Remove pan from oven and spoon juices from the bottom of the pan over the potatoes before serving.

Storage: Sweet potatoes are best served straight from the oven, but can be refrigerated for up to 2 days.

Serving Suggestion: Serve alongside Greek-Style Roast Chicken or Blackened Chicken Breast.

Variation: To make **Cinnamon Hasselback Sweet Potatoes**, replace the garlic slices with thinly sliced apples, use ground cinnamon instead of sage, and drizzle potatoes with honey instead of ghee before baking.

NUTRITION

Calories 194
Total Fat 10g
Saturated Fat 6g
Unsaturated Fat 3g
Cholesterol 25mg
Sodium 187mg
Carbohydrate 25g
Dietary Fiber 4g
Sugar 7g
Protein 3g

Grated cauliflower mimics the texture of rice in this **salty, savory stand-in** for the **Chinese takeout favorite.**

Cauliflower **Fried Rice**

 YIELD: **4 CUPS**   SERVING SIZE. **1 CUP**   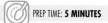 PREP TIME: **5 MINUTES**   COOK TIME: **15 MINUTES**

INGREDIENTS

5 cups cauliflower florets (about 1 medium head)

1 TB. olive oil

1 cup onion, chopped

1 cup carrots, chopped

1 TB. fresh ginger, peeled and minced

1 clove garlic, minced

3 green onions, chopped

1 TB. coconut aminos

1 TB. **Worcestershire Sauce**

SPECIAL TOOLS

 FOOD PROCESSOR

METHOD

1 In a food processor fitted with a chopping blade, pulse cauliflower for 5 to 10 seconds or until it is finely grated and resembles rice.

2 In a large skillet over high heat, add olive oil, onion, carrots, ginger, and garlic. Cook for 5 minutes or until soft.

3 Add cauliflower, stir, and cook for 5 minutes undisturbed, allowing the cauliflower to brown. Stir contents, scraping any browned bits from the bottom, and cook for another 5 minutes undisturbed.

4 Remove pan from heat. Stir in green onions, coconut aminos, and Worcestershire Sauce until the "rice" is evenly coated.

Storage: Cauliflower rice is best served immediately.

Serving Suggestion: Serve as side dish with Broccoli Beef Stir-Fry or Pineapple Teriyaki Salmon.

Use a hot, dry pan. Let the cauliflower brown at the bottom of the pan to prevent it from releasing too much liquid, which can cause the "rice" to become mushy.

NUTRITION

Calories 105	Saturated Fat 1g	Cholesterol 0mg	Carbohydrate 17g	Sugar 7g
Total Fat 4g	Unsaturated Fat 4g	Sodium 189mg	Dietary Fiber 5g	Protein 3g

The **creamy texture** of this easy-to-prepare side dish makes it the perfect healthy, AIP-friendly **substitute for traditional mashed potatoes**.

Parsnip Purée

 YIELD: **1 CUP**   SERVING SIZE: **½ CUP**   PREP TIME: **5 MINUTES**   COOK TIME: **30 MINUTES**

INGREDIENTS

2 cups parsnips, peeled and chopped

1 clove garlic, peeled

2 TB. ghee

¼ cup light coconut milk

¼ tsp. smoked sea salt

SPECIAL TOOLS

 FOOD PROCESSOR

METHOD

1 In a medium saucepan, cover parsnips and garlic with water. Cover and boil for 20 minutes over high heat.

2 Drain the parsnips, reserving the cooking liquid.

3 In a food processor, combine cooked parsnips, garlic, ghee, coconut milk, ¼ cup reserved cooking liquid, and smoked sea salt. Process for 30 seconds or until smooth.

Storage: Store in the refrigerator for up to 1 week or in the freezer for up to 3 months.

Serving Suggestion: Serve as a warm side dish with Apple Cider Pork Chops or Homestyle Meatloaf Muffins.

Variation: To make **Rutabaga Purée,** substitute 2 cups chopped rutabaga for the parsnips.

NUTRITION

Calories 234	Saturated Fat 10g	Cholesterol 33mg	Carbohydrate 25g	Sugar 7g
Total Fat 15g	Unsaturated Fat 5g	Sodium 304mg	Dietary Fiber 6g	Protein 2g

The lightly sweet, earthy flavor of butternut squash is complemented by **creamy coconut milk and maple syrup** in this hearty side dish.

Coconut **Butternut Squash** Mash

 YIELD: **3 CUPS**   SERVING SIZE: **½ CUP**   PREP TIME: **10 MINUTES**   COOK TIME: **40 MINUTES**

INGREDIENTS

1 medium butternut squash, cut in half lengthwise and seeds removed

3 TB. ghee

¼ cup light coconut milk

2 TB. plus 1 tsp. maple syrup

¼ tsp. sea salt

⅛ tsp. cinnamon

SPECIAL TOOLS

 FOOD PROCESSOR

METHOD

1 Preheat oven to 375°F (190°C).

2 Line a baking sheet with foil. Place butternut squash halves flesh side down. Bake for 30 to 40 minutes or until fork tender.

3 Scoop butternut squash out of the skin and place in a food processor.

4 Add ghee, coconut milk, maple syrup, and sea salt. Process for 30 seconds or until smooth.

5 Scoop into a serving dish and sprinkle with cinnamon.

Storage: Store in the refrigerator for up to 3 days or freeze for up to 3 months.

Variation: To make **Maple Sweet Potato Mash**, replace butternut squash with 4 cups peeled and chopped sweet potatoes.

NUTRITION

| Calories 124 | Saturated Fat 4g | Cholesterol 17mg | Carbohydrate 16g | Sugar 7g |
| Total Fat 7g | Unsaturated Fat 2g | Sodium 86mg | Dietary Fiber 3g | Protein 1g |

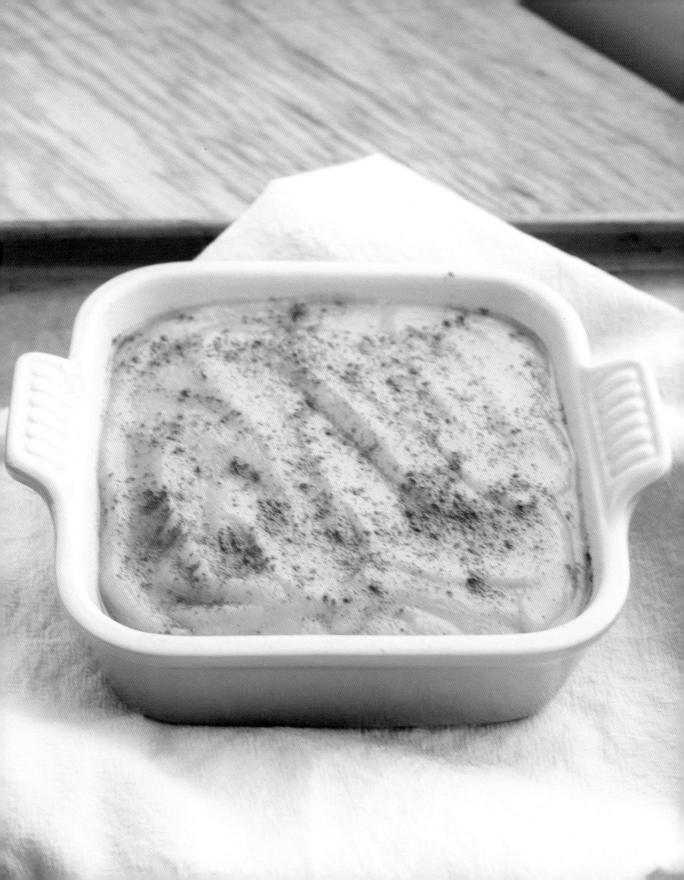

Marinating portobello mushrooms before grilling gives them a crispy, charred exterior and a juicy interior **packed with flavors of garlic and fresh thyme**.

Balsamic Grilled
Portobello Mushrooms

 YIELD: **4 MUSHROOMS**   SERVING SIZE: **1 MUSHROOM**   PREP TIME: **35 MINUTES**   COOK TIME: **8 MINUTES**

INGREDIENTS

¼ cup balsamic vinegar

¼ cup olive oil

2 TB. lemon juice

2 tsp. fresh thyme, chopped

4 garlic cloves, minced

3 portobello mushroom caps

SPECIAL TOOLS

 GRILL OR GRILL PAN

METHOD

1 In a small bowl, whisk together balsamic vinegar, olive oil, lemon juice, thyme, and garlic cloves.

2 Place mushroom caps in a large zipper-lock plastic bag.

3 Pour marinade over mushrooms, massaging it into the mushrooms to ensure they are well coated.

4 Refrigerate for at least 30 minutes or as long as overnight.

5 Heat a well-greased grill or grill pan over high heat. Grill mushroom for 4 minutes, flip, and cook for another 4 minutes.

Storage: Mushrooms are best served hot off the grill, but can be stored in the refrigerator for 2 days.

Serving Suggestion: Serve as a side dish with New Orleans Barbecue Shrimp, or chop and toss with Herbed Baked Spaghetti Squash.

NUTRITION

Calories 158

Total Fat 14g

Saturated Fat 2g

Unsaturated Fat 11g

Cholesterol 0mg

Sodium 45mg

Carbohydrate 8g

Dietary Fiber 1g

Sugar 2g

Protein 2g

Grilled onions bring a welcome **sweet-and-savory flavor** to almost any dish, making them a **versatile and delicious topping**.

Fool-Proof
Caramelized Onions

 YIELD: **1 CUP**   SERVING SIZE: **¼ CUP**   PREP TIME: **2 MINUTES**   COOK TIME: **20 MINUTES**

INGREDIENTS

2 cups yellow onion, thinly sliced
(1 large onion)

1 TB. olive oil

2 TB. vegetable broth

METHOD

1 Heat a skillet over medium-high heat. Add onions and olive oil. Cook onions for 10 minutes until soft and beginning to brown on the bottom of the pan.

2 Add 1 tablespoon vegetable broth, scraping up any caramelized bits from the bottom of the pan.

3 Cook onions for another 5 minutes. As the onions caramelize, they will become a dark golden brown.

4 Add remaining 1 tablespoon vegetable broth. Stir and cook for another 5 minutes.

Storage: Onions are best served immediately but can be refrigerated for up to 2 days.

Serving Suggestion: Serve onions atop Middle Eastern Bison Burgers, Apple Cider Pork Chops, or Orange Pulled Pork Carnitas.

> Don't worry about the onions sticking to the pan. Adding the vegetable broth will release the caramelized brown bits and allow the onions to stay moist while cooking.

NUTRITION

Calories 46	Saturated Fat 0g	Cholesterol 0mg	Carbohydrate 4g	Sugar 2g
Total Fat 3g	Unsaturated Fat 3g	Sodium 24mg	Dietary Fiber 1g	Protein 0g

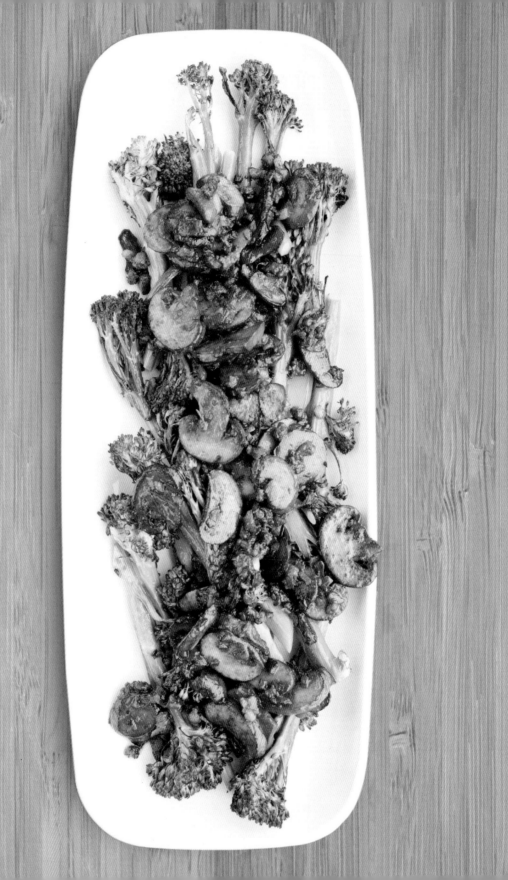

Broccolini has a milder, more delicate flavor than broccoli. In this recipe it is topped with the **smoky, savory flavors of pancetta, mushrooms, and garlic**.

Roasted Broccolini with
White Wine Mushrooms

 YIELD: **4 CUPS**   SERVING SIZE: **1 CUP**   PREP TIME: **10 MINUTES**   COOK TIME: **25 MINUTES**

INGREDIENTS

2 bunches broccolini, leaves removed and ends trimmed

1 TB. olive oil

1 TB. bacon fat

¼ cup shallots, chopped

1 clove garlic, minced

8 oz. (225g) cremini mushrooms, sliced

2 oz. (55g) pancetta, chopped

¼ cup dry white wine

METHOD

1 Preheat oven to 400°F (200°C). Line a baking sheet with foil.

2 Place broccolini on baking sheet. Drizzle with olive oil and massage oil into vegetables until well coated. Roast for 10 minutes.

3 In a large skillet over medium-high heat, combine bacon fat, shallots, garlic, mushrooms, and pancetta. Sauté for 10 minutes or until vegetables are tender.

4 Deglaze pan with wine and allow alcohol to cook off for another 2 to 5 minutes.

5 Remove broccolini from oven and transfer to a serving dish. Spoon white wine mushroom sauce over broccolini.

Storage: Broccolini is best served immediately, but can be stored in the refrigerator for up to 3 days.

Serving Suggestion: Serve as a side dish with Lemon-Stuffed Sea Bass or Bacon-Wrapped Scallops.

NUTRITION

Calories 186

Total Fat 13g

Saturated Fat 3g

Unsaturated Fat 5g

Cholesterol 13mg

Sodium 128mg

Carbohydrate 10g

Dietary Fiber 3g

Sugar 2g

Protein 6g

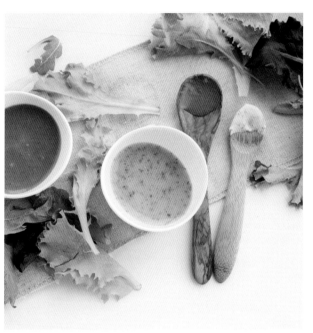

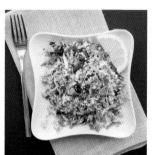

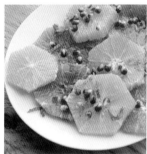

CHAPTER 7
Salads
& Dressings

Sweet Red Raspberry Vinaigrette

 YIELD: **1¼ CUP**   SERVING SIZE: **2 TB.**   PREP TIME: **2 MINUTES**   COOK TIME: **0 MINUTES**

INGREDIENTS

2 cups fresh raspberries

½ cup olive oil

2 TB. honey

3 TB. balsamic vinegar

3 TB. lemon juice

¼ tsp. sea salt

SPECIAL TOOLS

 FOOD PROCESSOR

METHOD

1 In a food processor, combine raspberries, olive oil, honey, balsamic vinegar, lemon juice, and salt.

2 Process for 30 seconds or until smooth. Transfer to an airtight container.

Storage: Store in an airtight container in the refrigerator for up to 1 week.

Serving Suggestion: Serve over Caribbean Chicken Salad or toss with mixed greens and serve alongside Maple Balsamic Glazed Salmon.

NUTRITION

Calories **128**
Total Fat **11g**
Saturated Fat **1g**
Unsaturated Fat **9g**
Cholesterol **0mg**
Sodium **61mg**
Carbohydrate **8g**
Dietary Fiber **2g**
Sugar **5g**
Protein **0g**

Cilantro Lime Vinaigrette

 YIELD: **1 CUP**   SERVING SIZE: **2 TB.**   PREP TIME: **5 MINUTES**   COOK TIME: **0 MINUTES**

INGREDIENTS

1 clove garlic, peeled

3 TB. lime juice

3 TB. orange juice

2 TB. honey

1 tsp. fresh ginger, peeled and minced

1 TB. cilantro, chopped

¼ cup olive oil

⅛ tsp. sea salt

SPECIAL TOOLS

 FOOD PROCESSOR

METHOD

1 In a food processor, combine garlic, lime juice, orange juice, honey, ginger, cilantro, olive oil, and sea salt.

2 Process for 30 seconds or until smooth. Transfer to an airtight container.

Storage: Store in an airtight container in the refrigerator for up to 1 week.

Serving Suggestion: Serve with Caribbean Chicken Salad or Citrus Mint Salad.

NUTRITION

Calories **81**
Total Fat **7g**
Saturated Fat **1g**
Unsaturated Fat **6g**
Cholesterol **0mg**
Sodium **37mg**
Carbohydrate **6g**
Dietary Fiber **0g**
Sugar **5g**
Protein **0g**

Cilantro Lime Vinaigrette

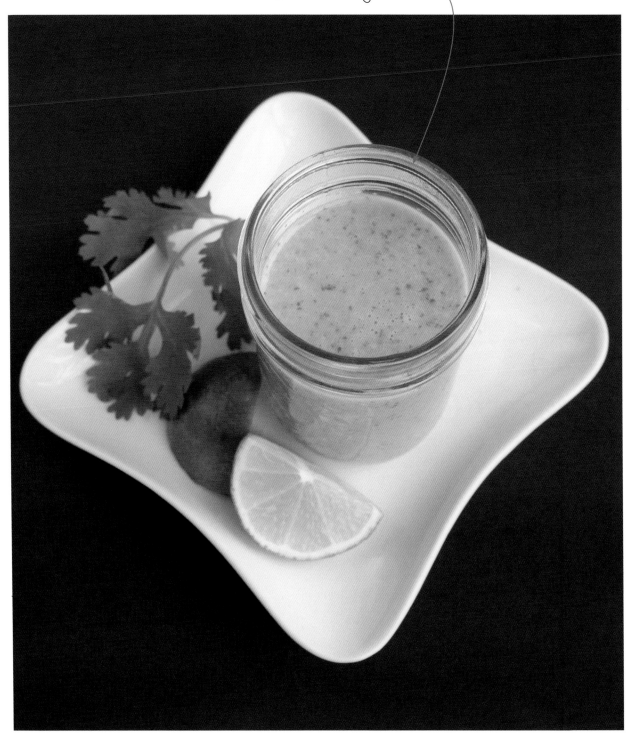

Creamy **Balsamic Dressing**

 YIELD: **2 CUPS**   SERVING SIZE: **2 TB.**   PREP TIME: **5 MINUTES**   COOK TIME: **0 MINUTES**

INGREDIENTS

⅓ cup balsamic vinegar

⅔ cup olive oil

¼ cup light coconut milk

¾ tsp. sea salt

¼ cup maple syrup

2 cloves garlic, peeled

SPECIAL TOOLS

 FOOD PROCESSOR

METHOD

1 In a food processor, combine balsamic vinegar, olive oil, coconut milk, salt, maple syrup, and garlic cloves.

2 Process for 30 seconds or until smooth. Transfer to an airtight container.

Storage: Store in an airtight container or jar in the refrigerator for up to 1 week.

NUTRITION

Calories 98

Total Fat 9g

Saturated Fat 1g

Unsaturated Fat 8g

Cholesterol 0mg

Sodium 90mg

Carbohydrate 4g

Dietary Fiber 0g

Sugar 3g

Protein 0g

Creamy Curry Vinaigrette

 YIELD: **1 CUP**   SERVING SIZE: **2 TB.**   PREP TIME: **2 MINUTES**   COOK TIME: **0 MINUTES**

INGREDIENTS

1 cup light coconut milk

1 TB. honey

3 TB. lemon juice

2 tsp. **Seed-Free Curry Powder**

⅛ tsp. sea salt

SPECIAL TOOLS

 FOOD PROCESSOR

METHOD

1 In a food processor, combine coconut milk, honey, lemon juice, Seed-Free Curry Powder, and sea salt.

2 Process for 30 seconds or until smooth. Transfer to an airtight container.

Storage: Store in an airtight container or jar in the refrigerator for up to 1 week.

NUTRITION

Calories 30

Total Fat 2g

Saturated Fat 2g

Unsaturated Fat 0g

Cholesterol 0mg

Sodium 39mg

Carbohydrate 4g

Dietary Fiber 0g

Sugar 3g

Protein 0g

Coconut Cream **Ranch Dressing**

 YIELD: **2 CUPS**   SERVING SIZE: **2 TB.**   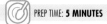 PREP TIME: **5 MINUTES**   COOK TIME: **0 MINUTES**

INGREDIENTS

1 (13.5-oz.; 400ml) can full fat coconut milk

2 cloves garlic, peeled

2 TB. apple cider vinegar

1 TB. lemon juice

¼ cup green onions

2 TB. parsley, chopped

1 tsp. dried basil

1 tsp. dried dill

¾ tsp. sea salt

METHOD

1 In a food processor, combine coconut milk, garlic, apple cider vinegar, lemon juice, green onions, parsley, basil, dill, and sea salt.

2 Process for 30 seconds or until smooth. Transfer to an airtight container.

Storage: Store in an airtight container or jar in the refrigerator for up to 1 week.

NUTRITION

Calories 75
Total Fat 7g
Saturated Fat 7g
Unsaturated Fat 0g
Cholesterol 0mg
Sodium 184mg
Carbohydrate 2g
Dietary Fiber 0g
Sugar 1g
Protein 0g

SPECIAL TOOLS

 FOOD PROCESSOR

Greek **Red Wine Vinaigrette**

 YIELD: **¾ CUP**   SERVING SIZE: **2 TB.**   PREP TIME: **5 MINUTES**   COOK TIME: **0 MINUTES**

INGREDIENTS

½ cup olive oil

2 TB. lemon juice

2 TB. red wine vinegar

1 clove garlic, peeled

1 tsp. dried oregano

¼ tsp. sea salt

METHOD

1 In a food processor, combine olive oil, lemon juice, red wine vinegar, garlic, oregano, and sea salt.

2 Process for 30 seconds or until smooth. Transfer to an airtight container.

Storage: Store in an airtight container or jar in the refrigerator for up to 1 week.

NUTRITION

Calories 163
Total Fat 18g
Saturated Fat 2g
Unsaturated Fat 15g
Cholesterol 0mg
Sodium 98mg
Carbohydrate 1g
Dietary Fiber 0g
Sugar 0g
Protein 0g

SPECIAL TOOLS

 FOOD PROCESSOR

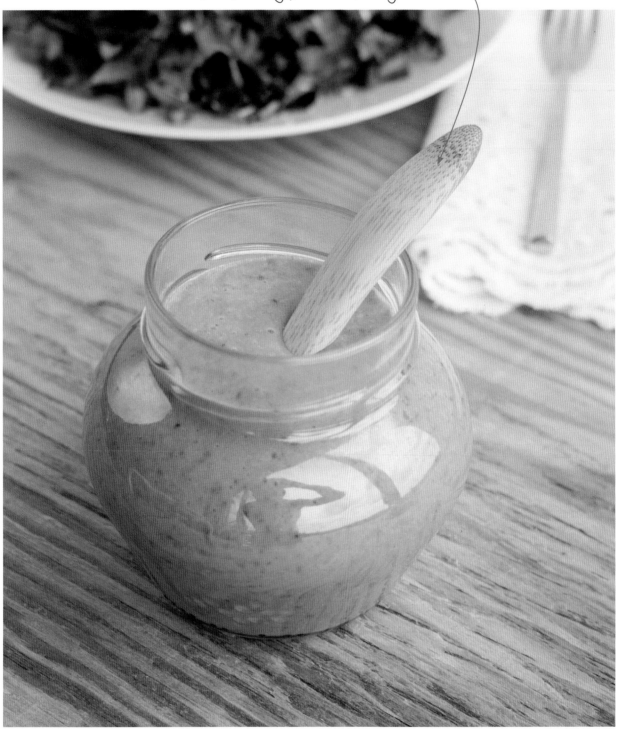

Strawberry Lemon Vinaigrette

Strawberry Lemon Vinaigrette

 YIELD: **2 CUPS**   SERVING SIZE: **2 TB.**   PREP TIME: **5 MINUTES**   COOK TIME: **0 MINUTES**

INGREDIENTS

3 cups strawberries, hulled

½ cup olive oil

¼ cup orange juice

1 TB. lemon juice

1 TB. balsamic vinegar

2 cloves garlic, peeled

1 tsp. lemon zest

⅛ tsp. sea salt

SPECIAL TOOLS

 FOOD PROCESSOR

METHOD

1 In a food processor, combine strawberries, olive oil, orange juice, lemon juice, balsamic vinegar, garlic, lemon zest, and sea salt.

2 Process for 30 seconds or until smooth. Transfer to an airtight container.

Storage: Store in an airtight container or jar in the refrigerator for up to 1 week.

NUTRITION

Calories 73

Total Fat 7g

Saturated Fat 1g

Unsaturated Fat 6g

Cholesterol 0mg

Sodium 16mg

Carbohydrate 3g

Dietary Fiber 1g

Sugar 2g

Protein 0g

Carrot Ginger Dressing

 YIELD: **2 CUPS**   SERVING SIZE: **2 TB.**   PREP TIME: **5 MINUTES**   COOK TIME: **20 MINUTES**

INGREDIENTS

½ cup carrot, peeled and chopped

½ cup water

2 TB. fresh ginger, minced

⅛ tsp. sea salt

2 TB. lemon juice

2 TB. apple cider vinegar

2 TB. honey

1 TB. olive oil

3 TB. light coconut milk

SPECIAL TOOLS

 FOOD PROCESSOR

METHOD

1 In a small saucepan, combine carrots and water. Bring to a boil. Reduce heat, cover, and simmer for 20 minutes or until fork-tender.

2 Transfer carrots and boiling water to food processor and add ginger, sea salt, lemon juice, apple cider vinegar, honey, olive oil, and coconut milk.

3 Process for 30 seconds or until smooth. Transfer to an airtight container.

Storage: Store in an airtight container or jar in the refrigerator for up to 1 week.

NUTRITION

Calories 20

Total Fat 1g

Saturated Fat 0g

Unsaturated Fat 1g

Cholesterol 0mg

Sodium 18mg

Carbohydrate 3g

Dietary Fiber 0g

Sugar 3g

Protein 0g

Celeriac, also known as celery root, has a **mild celery flavor** and crunchy texture that pairs well with **savory herbs and a sweet citrus dressing**.

Apple Currant **Celeriac Slaw**

 YIELD: **5 CUPS**   SERVING SIZE: **1¼ CUP**   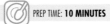 PREP TIME: **10 MINUTES**   COOK TIME: **0 MINUTES**

INGREDIENTS

4 cups celeriac, peeled and quartered (1 large bulb)

3 cups apple, peeled and quartered (1½ large apples)

1 TB. orange juice

Juice and zest of 1 lemon

⅛ tsp. sea salt

1 TB. fresh thyme, chopped

2 TB. fresh basil, chopped

½ cup dried currants, or raisins

SPECIAL TOOLS

 FOOD PROCESSOR

METHOD

1 Fit food processor with a shredding disc attachment. Feed celeriac and apple quarters into machine to grate.

2 In a small bowl, combine orange juice, lemon juice, lemon zest, and salt to make the dressing.

3 In a large bowl, combine grated celeriac and apple mixture with thyme, basil, and currants.

4 Pour dressing over slaw and toss to combine. Let sit for 5 minutes before serving.

Storage: Slaw is best enjoyed immediately.

Serving Suggestion: Serve as a side dish with Blackened Chicken Breast or Lemon-Stuffed Sea Bass.

> Celeriac is a variety of celery cultivated for its edible roots. This turnip-sized root has a knobby outer surface and smooth, white flesh with a mild, celery-like flavor.

NUTRITION

| Calories 171 | Saturated Fat 0g | Cholesterol 0mg | Carbohydrate 42g | Sugar 25g |
| Total Fat 0g | Unsaturated Fat 0g | Sodium 231mg | Dietary Fiber 6g | Protein 3g |

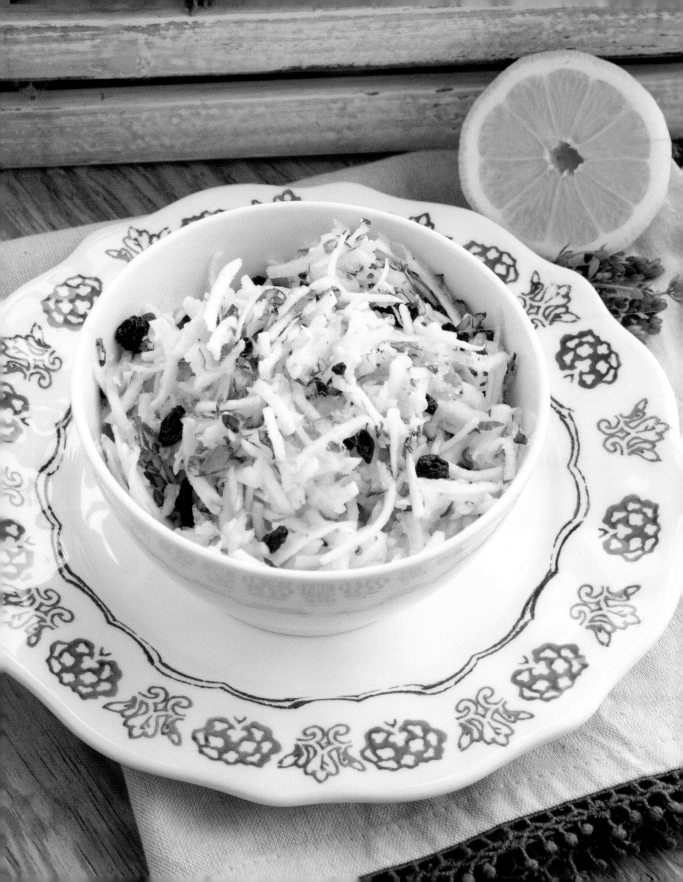

Put a **Mediterranean twist on a traditional favorite** with this unique tuna salad featuring plenty of crunchy, fresh vegetables and a **tangy avocado mayo**.

Mediterranean **Tuna Salad**

 YIELD: **8 CUPS**   SERVING SIZE: **1 CUP**   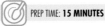 PREP TIME: **15 MINUTES**   CHILL TIME: **15 MINUTES**

INGREDIENTS

4 (6-oz; 170g) cans albacore tuna, drained

1 (14-oz; 395g) can artichoke hearts, drained and chopped

½ cup celery, chopped

½ cup cucumber, chopped

¾ cup green olives, pitted and chopped

1 cup red onion, chopped

¼ cup parsley, chopped

¼ cup fresh basil, chopped

1 tsp. dried oregano

½ cup **Basic Avocado "Mayo"**

½ tsp. sea salt

METHOD

1 In a large bowl, combine tuna, artichoke hearts, celery, cucumber, green olives, red onion, parsley, basil, oregano, Basic Avocado "Mayo," and sea salt. Gently stir until well mixed.

2 Refrigerate salad for 15 minutes before serving to allow flavors to come together.

Storage: Salad can be stored in the refrigerator for up to 3 days.

Serving Suggestion: Serve over a bed of mixed greens or crunchy romaine lettuce.

NUTRITION

Calories 192	Saturated Fat 2g	Cholesterol 13mg	Carbohydrate 6g	Sugar 1g
Total Fat 10g	Unsaturated Fat 3g	Sodium 832mg	Dietary Fiber 3g	Protein 18g

Guacamole meets chicken salad in this creamy combination of avocado, shredded chicken, and crunchy cucumber.

Avocado **Chicken Salad**

 YIELD: **6 CUPS**   SERVING SIZE: **1 CUP**   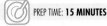 PREP TIME: **15 MINUTES**   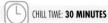 CHILL TIME: **30 MINUTES**

INGREDIENTS

4 cups cooked chicken breast, chopped

1 cup cucumber, finely chopped

1 cup red onion, finely chopped

1 clove garlic, minced

Juice of 1½ limes

¼ cup cilantro, chopped

2 avocados, mashed

½ tsp. sea salt

METHOD

1 In a large mixing bowl, combine chicken, cucumber, red onion, garlic, lime juice, cilantro, mashed avocado, and sea salt. Gently stir until well mixed.

2 Refrigerate salad for 30 minutes before serving to allow flavors to come together.

Storage: Salad can be stored in the refrigerator for up to 3 days.

Serving Suggestion: Serve salad over a bed of mixed greens, as a dip with chopped veggies, or alongside Rosemary Sweet Potato Chips or Crispy Cinnamon Apple Chips for a quick snack.

NUTRITION

Calories 283	Saturated Fat 2g	Cholesterol 79mg	Carbohydrate 7g	Sugar 2g
Total Fat 13g	Unsaturated Fat 2g	Sodium 221mg	Dietary Fiber 3g	Protein 38g

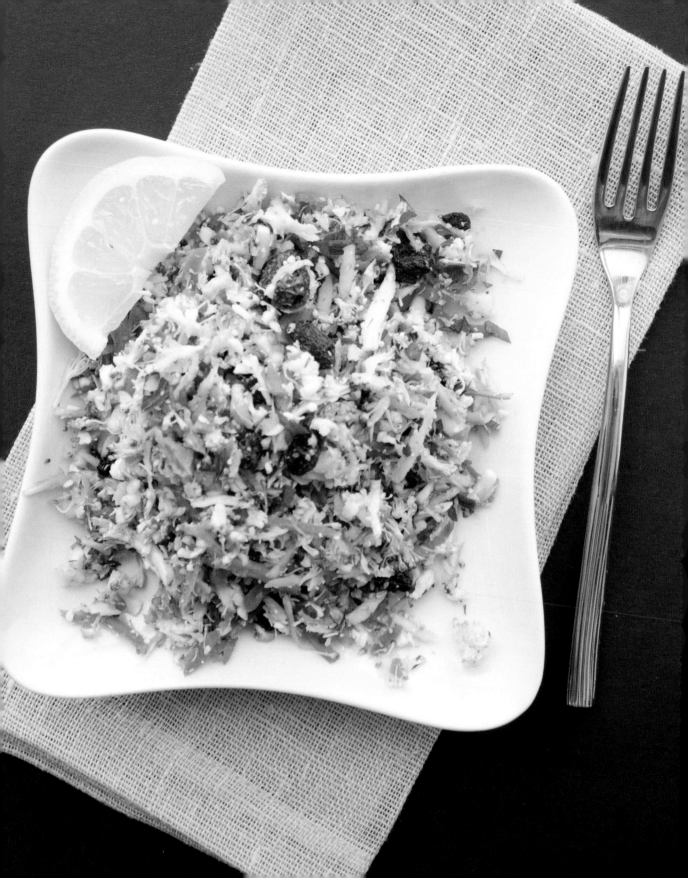

Cruciferous vegetables give this salad a **crunchy** texture, while the raisins and pineapple juice offer a **subtle hint of sweetness**.

Shaved **Broccoli and Cauliflower** Slaw

 YIELD: **12 CUPS**   SERVING SIZE: **2 CUPS**   PREP TIME: **10 MINUTES**   CHILL TIME: **20 MINUTES**

INGREDIENTS

8 cups broccoli florets

6 cups cauliflower florets

2½ cups carrots, peeled and roughly chopped

2 cups raisins

1 cup parsley, chopped

½ cup lemon juice

½ cup pineapple juice

1 TB. lemon zest

¼ tsp. sea salt

SPECIAL TOOLS

 FOOD PROCESSOR

METHOD

1 Fit food processor with a shredding disk attachment. Feed broccoli into machine and pulse until finely shredded. Transfer to a large bowl.

2 Feed cauliflower into food processor to grate. Transfer to the large bowl with the broccoli.

3 Feed carrots into food processor, pulse until finely shredded, and add to bowl with broccoli and cauliflower. Stir to combine.

4 Add raisins and parsley to the vegetable mixture and stir to combine.

5 In a small bowl, whisk together lemon juice, pineapple juice, lemon zest, and salt. Pour dressing over slaw and toss to combine.

6 Refrigerate for 20 minutes before serving to allow for flavors to come together.

Storage: Slaw is best served immediately, but can be stored in the refrigerator for up to 2 days.

NUTRITION

| Calories 274 | Saturated Fat 0g | Cholesterol 0mg | Carbohydrate 67g | Sugar 42g |
| Total Fat 1g | Unsaturated Fat 0g | Sodium 199mg | Dietary Fiber 9g | Protein 8g |

This summer salad offers the **fresh citrus flavors** of orange and grapefruit complemented by **tart pomegranate seeds** and **refreshing mint**.

Citrus Mint Salad

 YIELD: **4 CUPS**   SERVING SIZE: **1 CUP**   PREP TIME: **5 MINUTES**   COOK TIME: **0 MINUTES**

INGREDIENTS

2 oranges, peeled and sliced

1 grapefruit, peeled and sliced

1 cup pomegranate seeds

2 TB. lime juice

2 TB. honey

1 TB. fresh mint leaves, chopped

METHOD

1 On large platter, arrange orange, grapefruit, and pomegranate seeds.

2 In a small bowl, whisk together lime juice and honey.

3 Drizzle dressing over fruit and garnish with mint leaves.

Storage: Salad can be refrigerated for up to 3 days.

To remove pomegranate seeds, cut the fruit into quarters, submerge in a bowl of water, and gently remove the seeds from the pith. The seeds will sink to the bottom and the pith will float to the top.

NUTRITION

Calories 133	Saturated Fat 0g	Cholesterol 0mg	Carbohydrate 33g	Sugar 23g
Total Fat 1g	Unsaturated Fat 0g	Sodium 3mg	Dietary Fiber 4g	Protein 2g

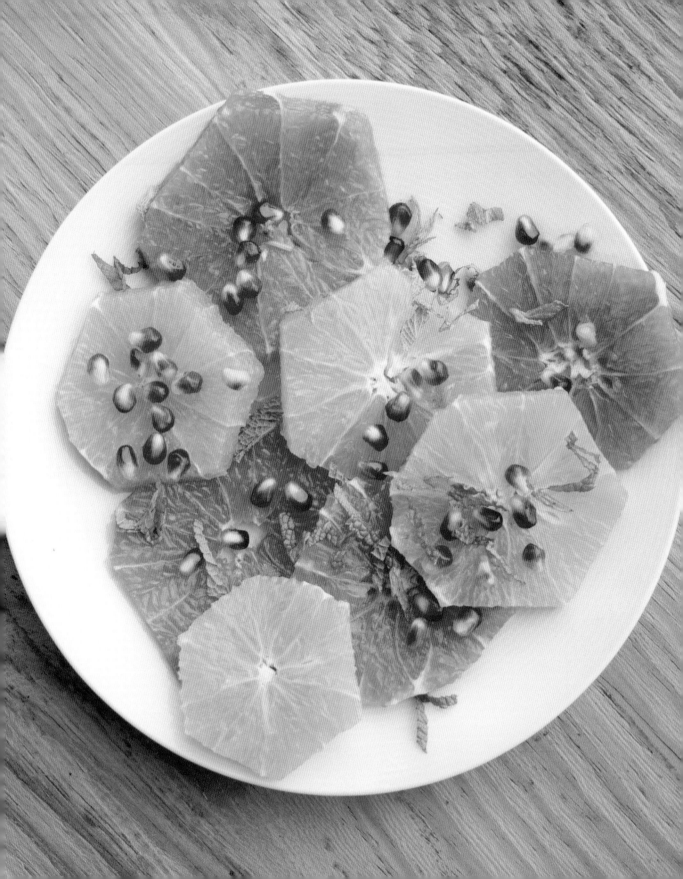

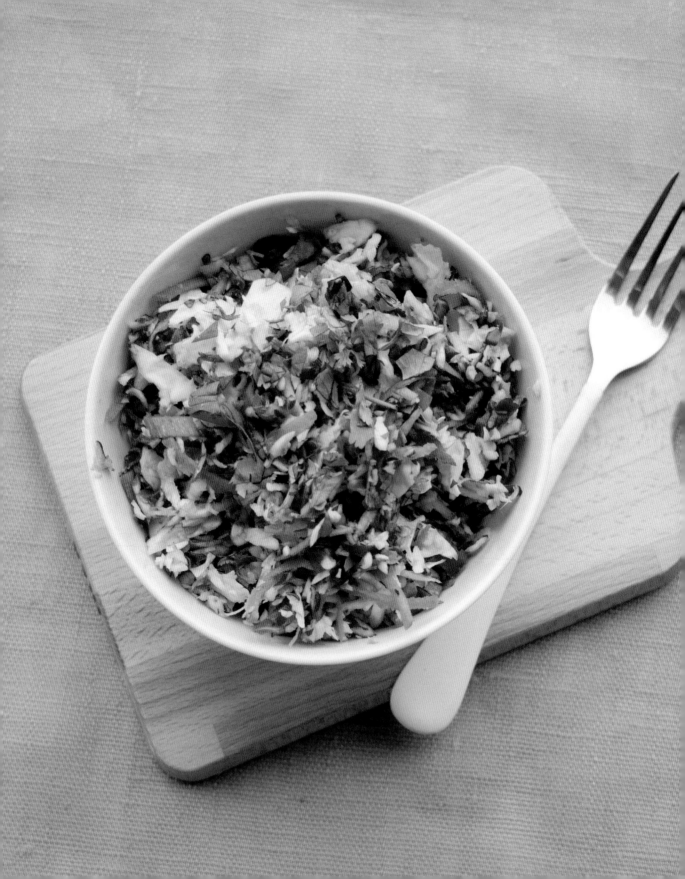

Vinegar-based slaws are lighter than traditional creamy ones. Packed with **tangy flavor**, this slaw makes a great side dish for any **backyard barbecue**.

Honey Vinegar
Tri-Colored Coleslaw

 YIELD: **9 CUPS**   SERVING SIZE: **1 CUP**   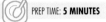 PREP TIME: **5 MINUTES**   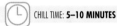 CHILL TIME: **5–10 MINUTES**

INGREDIENTS

3 cups red cabbage, shredded

3 cups green cabbage, shredded

2 carrots, peeled and shredded

½ cup green onions, chopped

2 TB. apple cider vinegar

4 TB. olive oil

1 clove garlic, minced

2 TB. honey

¼ tsp. sea salt

¼ cup cilantro, chopped

SPECIAL TOOLS

 FOOD PROCESSOR

METHOD

1 In a large bowl, combine red cabbage, green cabbage, carrots, and green onions.

2 In a small bowl, whisk together apple cider vinegar, olive oil, garlic, honey, and sea salt.

3 Pour dressing over cabbage mixture and toss to coat. Stir in cilantro.

4 Refrigerate for 5 to 10 minutes before serving to allow flavors to come together.

Storage: Slaw is best served immediately.

Serving Suggestion: Serve as a refreshing side dish with Pineapple Teriyaki Salmon or Middle Eastern Bison Burgers.

To quickly shred cabbage and carrots, use the shredding disk attachment that comes with most food processors. This attachment is often reversible to create fine or coarse shreds.

NUTRITION

Calories 109	Saturated Fat 1g	Cholesterol 0mg	Carbohydrate 12g	Sugar 8g
Total Fat 6g	Unsaturated Fat 0g	Sodium 103mg	Dietary Fiber 3g	Protein 1g

Fresh flavors of lemon juice and garlic join with creamy butternut squash and bright cranberries to create the **perfect warm winter salad**.

Classic Kale Salad

 YIELD: **2 CUPS**   SERVING SIZE: **1 CUP**   PREP TIME: **10 MINUTES**   COOK TIME: **20 MINUTES**

INGREDIENTS

2 cups butternut squash, peeled and cubed

1 TB. olive oil

⅛ tsp. sea salt

8 cups kale, stems removed and roughly chopped

2 TB. lemon juice

2 TB. **Greek Red Wine Vinaigrette**

1 TB. honey

⅓ cup dried cranberries

METHOD

1 Preheat oven to 375°F (190°C).

2 Line a baking sheet with foil. Spread butternut squash on baking sheet, drizzle with olive oil, and sprinkle with sea salt. Bake for 10 minutes.

3 While squash bakes, combine kale, lemon juice, and Greek Red Wine Vinaigrette in a large bowl. Using clean hands, massage dressing into kale leaves.

4 Remove squash from the oven. Flip and bake for another 5 minutes.

5 Remove squash from the oven, drizzle with honey, and bake for another 5 minutes.

6 Add squash and dried cranberries to kale and toss until combined.

Storage: Refrigerate for up to 2 days.

Serving Suggestion: Top warm kale salad with Greek-Style Roast Chicken, Maple Balsamic Glazed Salmon, or Lemon-Stuffed Sea Bass.

Massaging the lemon juice and dressing into the kale tenderizes the tough greens and minimizes the natural bitter flavors.

NUTRITION

Calories 218

Total Fat 9g

Saturated Fat 1g

Unsaturated Fat 7g

Cholesterol 0mg

Sodium 168mg

Carbohydrate 35g

Dietary Fiber 5g

Sugar 13g

Protein 5g

This crisp and refreshing salad showcases crunchy cucumber with a sweet-and-sour **honey vinegar dressing**.

Asian Cucumber Salad

 YIELD: **2 CUPS**   SERVING SIZE: **1 CUP**   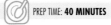 PREP TIME: **40 MINUTES**   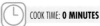 COOK TIME: **0 MINUTES**

INGREDIENTS

2 medium cucumbers, sliced into ¼-inch (6mm) slices

1 tsp. sea salt

¼ cup red onion, thinly sliced

1 TB. honey

1 TB. white wine vinegar

1 TB. sherry vinegar

METHOD

1 Place cucumbers in a colander over a bowl or sink. Sprinkle with sea salt and let drain for 30 minutes.

2 Remove cucumber slices from the colander and squeeze out excess water with paper towels or a clean dish towel.

3 In a large bowl, combine cucumbers and red onion.

4 In a small bowl, whisk together honey, white wine vinegar, and sherry vinegar.

5 Pour dressing over cucumber salad and toss to combine.

Storage: Cucumber salad is best enjoyed immediately.

Serving Suggestion: Serve cucumber salad as a side dish with Greek-Style Roast Chicken, Burgundy Lamb Kabobs, or Asian Turkey Lettuce Wraps.

Because cucumbers have a high water content, cucumber salads can often become soggy. Salting and draining the cucumbers removes excess water and allows them to absorb the tangy dressing.

NUTRITION

Calories 84	Saturated Fat 0g	Cholesterol 0mg	Carbohydrate 21g	Sugar 15g
Total Fat 0g	Unsaturated Fat 0g	Sodium 1,173mg	Dietary Fiber 2g	Protein 2g

This **all-American garden salad** varies slightly from the traditional version, but still features many of the classic ingredients of this **lunchtime favorite**.

Grilled Chicken **Cobb Salad**

 YIELD: **12 CUPS**   SERVING SIZE: **3 CUPS**   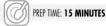 PREP TIME: **15 MINUTES**   COOK TIME: **10 MINUTES**

INGREDIENTS

3 (6-oz.; 170g) boneless, skinless chicken breasts

1 TB. olive oil

¼ tsp. sea salt

8 cups romaine lettuce, chopped

1 large avocado, chopped

½ cup parsley, chopped

6 slices bacon, cooked and chopped

2 cups cucumber, peeled and chopped

½ cup green onions, chopped

SPECIAL TOOLS

 GRILL OR GRILL PAN

METHOD

1 Place chicken breasts between two sheets of parchment paper. With a meat mallet, pound to an even thickness of ½ inch (1.25cm).

2 Brush both sides of chicken breasts with olive oil and season with sea salt.

3 Heat a grill or grill pan to medium-high heat. Place chicken breasts on the grill and cook until browned on the bottom, about 3 to 5 minutes. Flip and cook until cooked through, about another 3 to 5 minutes.

4 Remove chicken from the grill and set aside to cool. When cool enough to touch, chop into bite-size pieces.

5 Place 2 cups romaine lettuce on each salad plate. Working in rows, top lettuce with avocado, parsley, bacon, cucumber, green onions, and chicken.

Storage: Salad is best served immediately.

Serving Suggestion: Top with Coconut Cream Ranch Dressing or Greek Red Wine Vinaigrette.

> For fast assembly, prep the chicken, bacon, and cucumber ahead of time and refrigerate until ready to use.

NUTRITION

Calories 325	Saturated Fat 5g	Cholesterol 53mg	Carbohydrate 12g	Sugar 3g
Total Fat 20g	Unsaturated Fat 10g	Sodium 736mg	Dietary Fiber 7g	Protein 28g

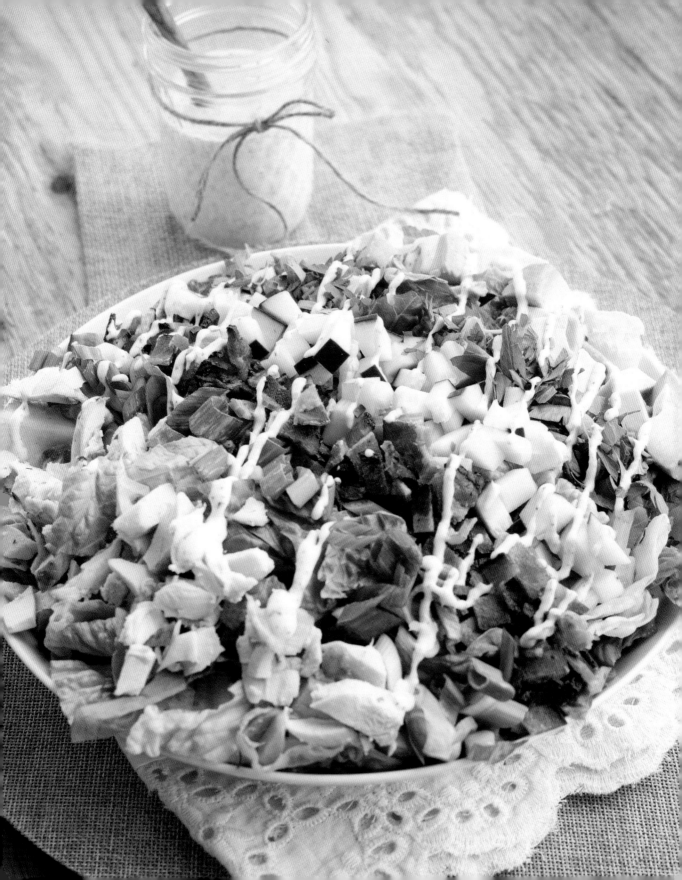

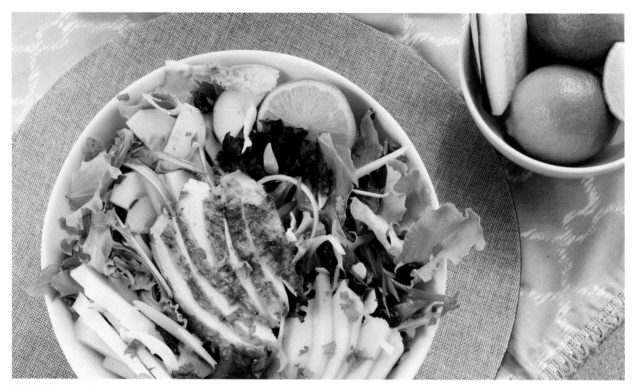

DIY Dressing

Making a basic homemade salad dressing is easy! Start by choosing one oil, one acid, one sweet or savory flavor, and one (or more) herb or spice.

Combine 3 parts oil to 1 part acid and mix and match other seasonings to taste. Start with 1 tablespoon sweet or savory flavor and 1 teaspoon of herb or spice and add more to reach desired flavor.

3 PARTS	**1 PART**	**ADD TO TASTE**	
OIL Olive oil Coconut oil Avocado oil	**ACID** Red wine vinegar White wine vinegar Balsamic vinegar Apple cider vinegar Sherry vinegar Lemon juice Lime juice Orange juice	**SWEET OR SAVORY FLAVOR** Lemon zest **Worcestershire Sauce** Naturally sweetened jam Maple syrup Honey	**HERBS & SPICES** Thyme Rosemary Basil Dill Tarragon Chives Garlic Shallots Ginger

The **fresh tropical flavors** of mango and coconut pair perfectly with the refreshing texture of **jicama and cucumber** in this easy-to-assemble salad.

Caribbean Chicken Salad

 YIELD: **12 CUPS**   SERVING SIZE: **3 CUPS**   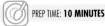 PREP TIME: **10 MINUTES**   COOK TIME: **10 MINUTES**

INGREDIENTS

3 (6-oz.; 170g) boneless, skinless chicken breasts

1 TB. olive oil

¼ tsp. sea salt

4 cups mixed greens

1 jicama, peeled and chopped

1 mango, peeled and sliced

1 cucumber, peeled and sliced

½ cup green onions, sliced

¼ cup unsweetened shredded coconut

¼ cup dried cranberries

SPECIAL TOOLS

 GRILL OR GRILL PAN

METHOD

1 Place chicken breasts between two sheets of parchment paper. With a meat mallet, pound to an even thickness of ½ inch (1.25cm).

2 Brush both sides of chicken breasts with olive oil and season with sea salt.

3 Heat grill or grill pan to medium-high heat. Place chicken breasts on grill and cook until browned on the bottom, about 3 to 5 minutes. Flip and cook until cooked through, about 3 to 5 minutes more.

4 Remove chicken from grill and let cool. When cool enough to touch, slice into strips.

5 In a large bowl, toss mixed greens, jicama, mango, cucumber, and green onions to combine.

6 Top salad with sliced chicken, shredded coconut, and cranberries.

Storage: Salad is best served immediately.

Serving Suggestion: Serve salad with Cilantro Lime Vinaigrette or Sweet Red Raspberry Vinaigrette.

Jicama is a bulbous tuber with crisp, white flesh. It tastes like a cross between a sweet pear and a starchy potato. Peeled and chopped, it can be used raw or cooked in soups and stir-fries.

NUTRITION

Calories 303

Total Fat 8g

Saturated Fat 3g

Unsaturated Fat 4g

Cholesterol 45g

Sodium 539mg

Carbohydrate 36g

Dietary Fiber 12g

Sugar 17g

Protein 25g

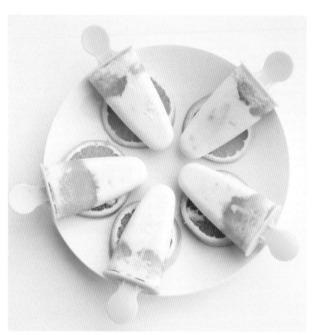
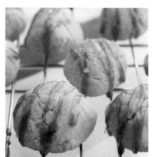
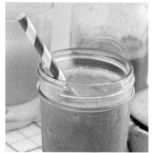

CHAPTER 8

Desserts
& Beverages

Enjoy the **buttery** flavors of **caramel** without the heavy cream. This **decadent, salt-kissed sauce** is the perfect accompaniment to any dessert.

Sea Salt **Caramel Sauce**

 YIELD: **¾ CUP**   SERVING SIZE: **1½ TB.**   PREP TIME: **5 MINUTES**   COOK TIME: **10 MINUTES**

INGREDIENTS

¼ cup coconut cream

¼ cup honey

2 TB. coconut sugar

1 TB. vanilla extract

Dash sea salt

1 TB. ghee

METHOD

1 In a small saucepan over medium heat, bring coconut cream, honey, and coconut sugar to a boil.

2 Add vanilla extract and sea salt and reduce heat to low.

3 Simmer for 5 minutes, stirring frequently.

4 Remove from heat and stir in ghee until melted and combined.

Storage: Enjoy warm immediately, or refrigerate for up to 1 month.

Serving Suggestion: Drizzle Sea Salt Caramel Caramel Sauce over fresh fruit, serve as a dip with Crispy Cinnamon Apple Chips, or use to make Caramel Coconut Macaroons.

To make your own coconut cream, refrigerate a can of full-fat coconut milk overnight. The thick cream will rise to the top; you can then separate it from the remaining liquid portion.

NUTRITION

Calories 78	Saturated Fat 2g	Cholesterol 4mg	Carbohydrate 12g	Sugar 12g
Total Fat 3g	Unsaturated Fat 10g	Sodium 22mg	Dietary Fiber 0g	Protein 0g

When whipped with a little sweetener, **coconut cream is transformed** into a **light, fluffy,** and **delicious** dessert topping.

Coconut Whipped Cream

 YIELD: **1½ CUPS**   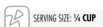 SERVING SIZE: **¼ CUP**   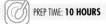 PREP TIME: **10 HOURS**   COOK TIME: **NONE**

INGREDIENTS

1 (13.5-oz; 400ml) can full-fat coconut milk

¼ cup coconut water

3 TB. maple syrup

SPECIAL TOOLS

 MIXER

METHOD

1 Place the can of full-fat coconut milk in the refrigerator and chill overnight.

2 Chill a metal mixing bowl in the freezer for 5 minutes.

3 Scoop coconut cream out of can and into the chilled bowl, leaving behind coconut water that has settled to the bottom of the can.

4 Whip coconut cream with electric mixer on low until creamy (about 1 minute).

5 Add coconut water and maple syrup and continue whipping until light and fluffy (about 2 minutes).

Storage: Store in the refrigerator for up to 3 days.

Serving Suggestion: Serve on top of fresh berries or Pumpkin Spice Ice Cream.

NUTRITION

Calories 146	Saturated Fat 10g	Cholesterol 0mg	Carbohydrate 9g	Sugar 8g
Total Fat 12g	Unsaturated Fat 0g	Sodium 16mg	Dietary Fiber 0g	Protein 0g

With sweet, creamy banana and a rich, chocolate-like coating, this **melt-in-your-mouth dessert** will satisfy your sweet tooth in **one small bite.**

Frozen **Banana Bites**

 YIELD: **16 PIECES**   SERVING SIZE: **2 PIECES**   PREP TIME: **12 HOURS**   CHILL TIME: **12 HOURS**

INGREDIENTS

1 large banana, peeled and sliced into ½-inch (1.25cm) pieces

½ cup coconut oil

1 TB. carob powder

2 TB. maple syrup

SPECIAL TOOLS

 MIXER

METHOD

1 Place sliced banana pieces on a large plate or other freezer-safe flat surface lined with parchment paper. Cover with foil and freeze for 12 hours until frozen solid.

2 In a large bowl, beat coconut oil on medium-low with an electric mixer for 2 minutes or until creamy and smooth.

3 Add carob powder and maple syrup and beat for another 2 minutes or until contents are well combined.

4 Remove frozen banana pieces from the freezer. Dip each piece into sauce and return to the parchment paper. Continue dipping banana pieces one at a time until all pieces are covered.

5 Freeze for at least 12 hours until coating is frozen.

Storage: Store in the freezer for up to 3 months.

Serving Suggestion: For added texture and crunch, sprinkle Frozen Banana Bites with unsweetened shredded coconut before serving.

NUTRITION

Calories **152**
Total Fat **14g**
Saturated Fat **12g**
Unsaturated Fat **2g**
Cholesterol **0mg**
Sodium **1mg**
Carbohydrate **9g**
Dietary Fiber **1g**
Sugar **6g**
Protein **0g**

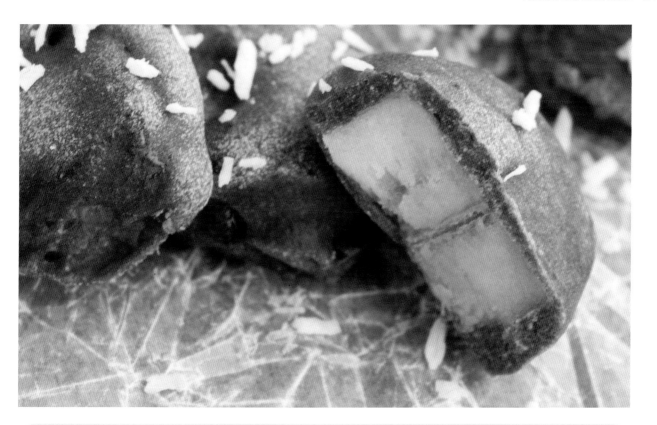

A Very Versatile Oil

Coconut oil is extracted from coconut meat and is naturally a semi-soft solid at room temperature. It can be melted to a liquid over heat or refrigerated to become hard and solid. The versatility of its consistency allows you to melt the oil for a recipe, form it as needed, and then set it with refrigeration.

Coconut oil melts to a liquid
very easily and has many uses.

Enjoy the **fall flavors of pumpkin pie** with this **easy frozen treat** featuring the warm spice of cinnamon and the sweetness of maple syrup.

Pumpkin Spice Ice Cream

 YIELD: **3 CUPS**   SERVING SIZE: **½ CUP**   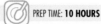 PREP TIME: **10 HOURS**   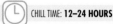 CHILL TIME: **12–24 HOURS**

INGREDIENTS

1 (13.5-oz; 400ml) can light coconut milk

½ cup Medjool dates, pitted (about 5 dates)

½ cup water

¼ cup plus 2 TB. pumpkin purée

2 TB. maple syrup

½ tsp. ground cinnamon

SPECIAL TOOLS

 BLENDER

METHOD

1 In a freezer-safe container, whisk coconut milk until smooth and creamy. Cover and freeze 8 to 10 hours or overnight.

2 Soak Medjool dates in warm water for 5 minutes until soft. Drain.

3 In a high-speed blender, combine coconut milk, drained Medjool dates, water, pumpkin purée, maple syrup, and cinnamon. Blend until smooth.

4 Return coconut mixture to freezer for 12 to 24 hours until frozen.

Storage: Store in the freezer for up to 3 months.

Serving Suggestion: When ready to serve, remove ice cream from the freezer and let it sit out for 5 to 10 minutes until soft. Serve with a dollop of Coconut Whipped Cream.

NUTRITION

Calories 120	Saturated Fat 4g	Cholesterol 0mg	Carbohydrate 22g	Sugar 19g
Total Fat 4g	Unsaturated Fat 0g	Sodium 2mg	Dietary Fiber 2g	Protein 1g

Refreshing and summery, this sorbet combines **ripe peaches** and **creamy coconut milk** with **tart white grape juice.**

Coconut Peach Sorbet

 YIELD: **3 CUPS**   SERVING SIZE: ⅓ **CUP**   PREP TIME: **5 MINUTES**   COOK TIME: **NONE**

INGREDIENTS

4 cups frozen peaches

½ cup light coconut milk

½ cup white grape juice

SPECIAL TOOLS

 BLENDER

METHOD

1 In a high-speed blender, combine peaches, coconut milk, and white grape juice.

2 Blend on high until combined and smooth. Sorbet will be ready to eat immediately.

Storage: Freeze for up to 3 months.

Serving Suggestion: If sorbet has been in the freezer, let it sit at room temperature for 5 to 10 minutes to soften before serving.

A high-speed blender is key to making fresh sorbet from frozen fruit. Use a wooden spoon to push ingredients toward the blade between rounds of blending until the sorbet is a smooth consistency.

NUTRITION

| Calories 133 | Saturated Fat 2g | Cholesterol 0mg | Carbohydrate 25g | Sugar 19g |
| Total Fat 2g | Unsaturated Fat 0g | Sodium 6mg | Dietary Fiber 3g | Protein 1g |

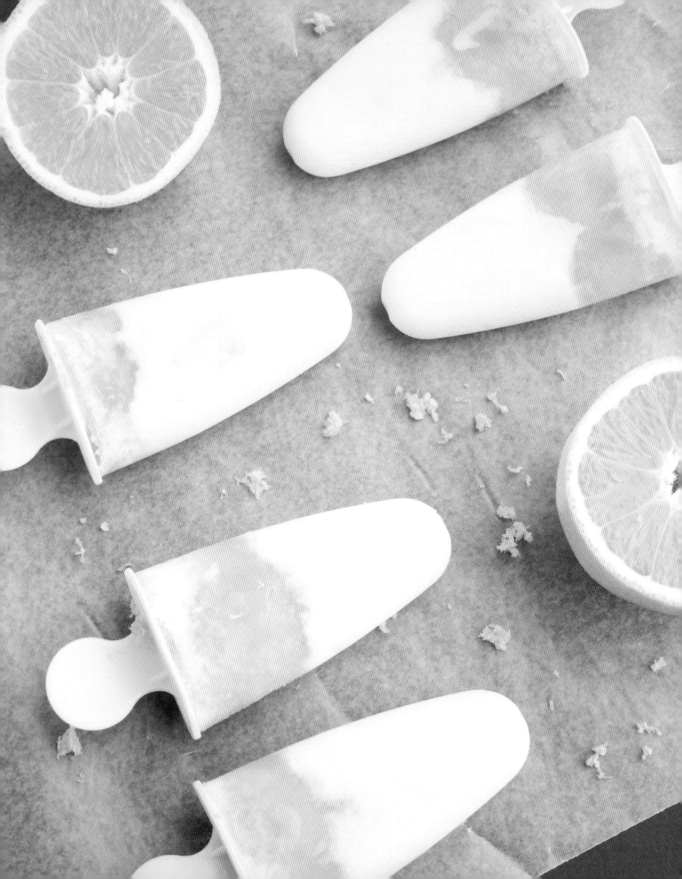

This **dairy-free frozen fruit pop** combines creamy coconut milk and freshly squeezed orange juice for an AIP twist on the **classic summer favorite.**

Orange **Creamsicle**

 YIELD: **12 FROZEN FRUIT POPS**   SERVING SIZE: **1 FROZEN FRUIT POP**   PREP TIME: **20 MINUTES**   CHILL TIME: **12–24 HOURS**

INGREDIENTS

- 1 (13.5-oz; 400ml) can light coconut milk
- 4 TB. maple syrup
- 1 cup freshly squeezed orange juice
- 1 TB. orange zest

SPECIAL TOOLS

 ICE POP MOLDS

METHOD

1 In a large bowl, whisk together coconut milk and 2 tablespoons maple syrup until smooth.

2 Pour coconut mixture into ice pop mold, filling each mold halfway. Freeze for 10 minutes.

3 In a small bowl, whisk together orange juice, orange zest, and remaining 2 tablespoons maple syrup.

4 Remove coconut mixture from the freezer, pour orange juice mixture into the molds, and insert the sticks. Freeze for 12 to 24 hours or until frozen through.

Storage: Store in the freezer for up to 3 months.

Variation: To make Strawberry Banana Fruit Pops, replace orange juice mixture with 1 cup strawberry purée and ¼ cup chopped banana.

> Don't have an ice pop mold? Use plastic cups and wooden treat sticks instead.

NUTRITION

Calories 47	Saturated Fat 2g	Cholesterol 0mg	Carbohydrate 7g	Sugar 7g
Total Fat 2g	Unsaturated Fat 0g	Sodium 1mg	Dietary Fiber 0g	Protein 0g

This **cozy dessert** is a healthy alternative to baked apple pie and features all of the same **sweet and spicy autumn flavors**.

Warm Cinnamon Apples

 YIELD: **2 CUPS**   SERVING SIZE: **½ CUP** 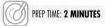 PREP TIME: **2 MINUTES**   COOK TIME: **20 MINUTES**

INGREDIENTS

1 TB. ghee

3 cups apples, peeled and chopped (about 2 medium apples)

½ cup raisins

2 TB. maple syrup

1 tsp. vanilla extract

¼ tsp. cinnamon

METHOD

1 In a large skillet, heat ghee over medium heat.

2 Add apples, raisins, maple syrup, vanilla extract, and cinnamon. Stir to combine.

3 Cover and cook for 20 minutes or until apples are fork-tender.

Storage: Store in the refrigerator for up to 3 days.

Serving Suggestion: Serve with Coconut Whipped Cream or atop a Flourless Brownie for a warm, satisfying dessert.

NUTRITION

| Calories 168 | Saturated Fat 2g | Cholesterol 8mg | Carbohydrate 36g | Sugar 29g |
| Total Fat 4g | Unsaturated Fat 1g | Sodium 4mg | Dietary Fiber 3g | Protein 1g |

Frying bananas in coconut oil gives them a **crisp and caramelized** exterior with a **warm and creamy center**.

Honey Fried Bananas

 YIELD: **2 BANANAS**   SERVING SIZE: ½ **BANANA**   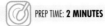 PREP TIME: **2 MINUTES**   COOK TIME: **5 MINUTES**

INGREDIENTS

½ cup warm water

1 TB. honey

2 TB. coconut oil

2 medium underripe bananas, peeled and sliced

⅛ tsp. cinnamon

METHOD

1 In a small bowl, whisk together warm water and honey.

2 Heat coconut oil in a large skillet over medium-high heat.

3 Add banana slices and fry for 2 minutes. Flip and fry for another 2 minutes or until bananas are a crisp golden brown on both sides.

4 Remove the pan from heat and pour honey-water mixture over bananas.

5 Sprinkle with cinnamon and let cool slightly before serving.

Storage: Fried bananas are best served immediately.

Serving Suggestion: Serve with Coconut Whipped Cream or atop Pumpkin Spice Ice Cream.

NUTRITION

Calories 127	Saturated Fat 6g	Cholesterol 0mg	Carbohydrate 18g	Sugar 12g
Total Fat 7g	Unsaturated Fat 0g	Sodium 1mg	Dietary Fiber 2g	Protein 1g

With a **crunchy fudge-like topping**, creamy mint center, and chewy, chocolaty crust, these frozen dessert bars are **sure to please** any chocolate lover.

Chocolaty Mint Bars

 YIELD: **9 BARS**   SERVING SIZE: **1 BAR**   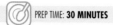 PREP TIME: **30 MINUTES**   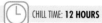 CHILL TIME: **12 HOURS**

INGREDIENTS

1 cup dates, pitted

1 cup shredded coconut

¼ cup carob powder

¼ cup + 1 TB. + 1 tsp. maple syrup

½ cup coconut oil

1 avocado, skin and pit removed

1 banana, peeled

½ tsp. peppermint extract

¼ cup coconut butter

SPECIAL TOOLS

 FOOD PROCESSOR

NUTRITION

Calories **314**
Total Fat **20g**
Saturated Fat **17g**
Unsaturated Fat **1g**
Cholesterol **0mg**
Sodium **7mg**
Carbohydrate **40g**
Dietary Fiber **7g**
Sugar **32g**
Protein **2g**

METHOD

1 In a small bowl, soak dates in warm water for 5 minutes or until softened.

2 In a food processor, combine dates, shredded coconut, 2 TB. carob powder, 1 TB. maple syrup, and 1 TB. coconut oil. Process for 30 seconds, scraping down the sides as needed, until mixture begins to form a ball.

3 Line an 8x8-inch (20x20cm) baking sheet with parchment paper. Press coconut mixture into the bottom of the pan to create the crust layer. Place the pan in the freezer.

4 In a clean food processor, combine avocado, banana, ¼ cup maple syrup, 3 TB. coconut oil, and peppermint extract. Process for 30 seconds or until smooth and creamy.

5 Remove the baking pan from the refrigerator and spoon avocado filling on top of coconut crust. Spread until even. Place the pan back in the freezer.

6 In a small saucepan, combine coconut butter and ¼ cup coconut oil. Heat over low heat until melted. Remove from heat and stir in 1 tsp. maple syrup and 2 TB. carob powder until smooth.

7 Remove the pan from the freezer and pour chocolate fudge layer on top of avocado layer, tilting the pan to cover the entire surface.

8 Return the pan to the freezer and freeze overnight or until solid.

Storage: Store in the freezer for up to 3 weeks.

Variation: To make **Tart Raspberry Sorbet Bars,** replace banana with 2 cups fresh raspberries and omit peppermint extract.

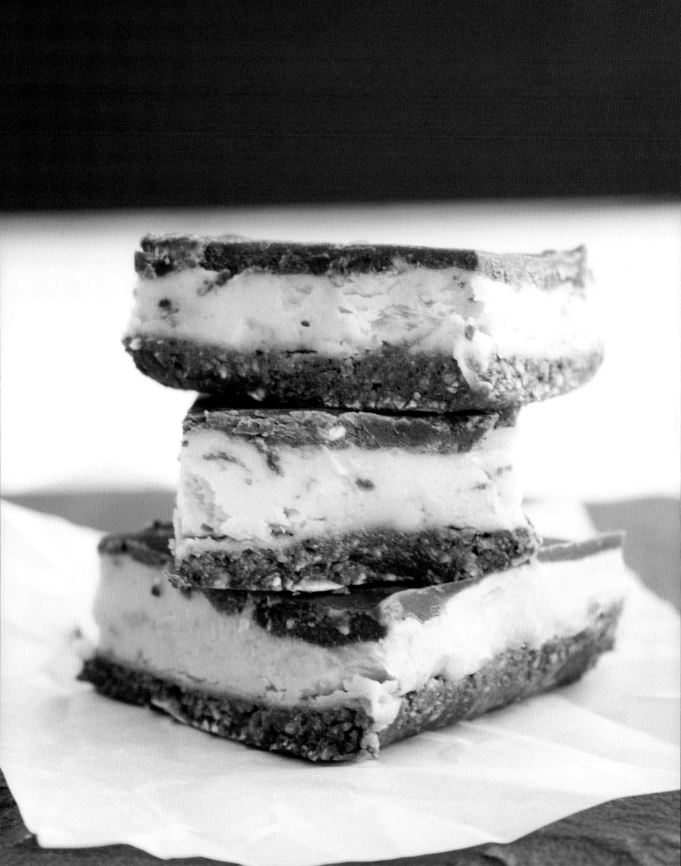

Coconut flour and carob powder lend a **rich, fudgey flavor,** while gelatin powder provides a cake-like texture for these **AIP-friendly brownies.**

Flourless **Brownies**

 YIELD: **12 BROWNIES**   SERVING SIZE: **1 BROWNIE**   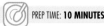 PREP TIME: **10 MINUTES**   COOK TIME: **30 MINUTES**

INGREDIENTS

⅓ cup plus 1 TB. coconut oil

½ cup unsweetened applesauce

¼ cup honey

1 tsp. vanilla extract

1 tsp. apple cider vinegar

3 TB. carob powder

¼ cup arrowroot powder

⅓ cup coconut flour

½ tsp. baking soda

¼ tsp. cinnamon

¼ tsp. sea salt

1 TB. gelatin powder

¼ cup water

SPECIAL TOOLS

 MIXER

METHOD

1 Preheat the oven to 350°F (180°C). Grease an 8×8-inch (20×20cm) pan with 1 tablespoon coconut oil.

2 In a large bowl, combine applesauce, remaining ⅓ cup coconut oil, honey, vanilla extract, and apple cider vinegar. Beat contents with an electric mixer for 30 seconds or until well combined.

3 In a small bowl, sift carob powder, arrowroot flour, coconut flour, baking soda, cinnamon, and sea salt.

4 In a small saucepan over low heat, combine gelatin powder and water. Whisk until dissolved. Cook over low heat for 1 to 2 minutes.

5 Meanwhile, add bowl of dry ingredients to bowl of wet ingredients and beat until combined.

6 Remove gelatin mixture from heat and whisk quickly until frothy. Fold gelatin mixture into brownie batter with a spatula.

7 Spread batter into the baking pan. Bake for 25 minutes or until toothpick inserted in center comes out clean. Cool in the pan for 10 minutes before cutting.

Storage: Store in the refrigerator for up to 1 week.

Serving Suggestion: Drizzle with Sea Salt Caramel Sauce or serve with Pumpkin Spice Ice Cream.

NUTRITION

Calories 121	Saturated Fat 12g	Cholesterol 0mg	Carbohydrate 15g	Sugar 9g
Total Fat 8g	Unsaturated Fat 1g	Sodium 108mg	Dietary Fiber 3g	Protein 2g

The **sweet banana, creamy avocado,** and **rich carob powder** in this recipe replicate the thick and frothy texture of a **chocolate milkshake**.

Banana Carob Shake

 YIELD: **2 CUPS**   SERVING SIZE: **1 CUP**   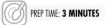 PREP TIME: **3 MINUTES**   COOK TIME: **NONE**

INGREDIENTS

1 cup kale leaves, stems removed

1 banana, peeled

¼ avocado, skin and pit removed

2 TB. carob powder

1 TB. honey

1 tsp. cinnamon

1 cup light coconut milk

½ cup water

10 to 12 ice cubes

METHOD

1 Combine kale, banana, avocado, carob powder, honey, cinnamon, coconut milk, water, and ice cubes in a blender.

2 Blend on high for 30 seconds or until smooth.

Storage: Shake is best enjoyed immediately.

SPECIAL TOOLS

 BLENDER

NUTRITION

Calories 210	Saturated Fat 9g	Cholesterol 0mg	Carbohydrate 43g	Sugar 24g
Total Fat 9g	Unsaturated Fat 0g	Sodium 50mg	Dietary Fiber 12g	Protein 2g

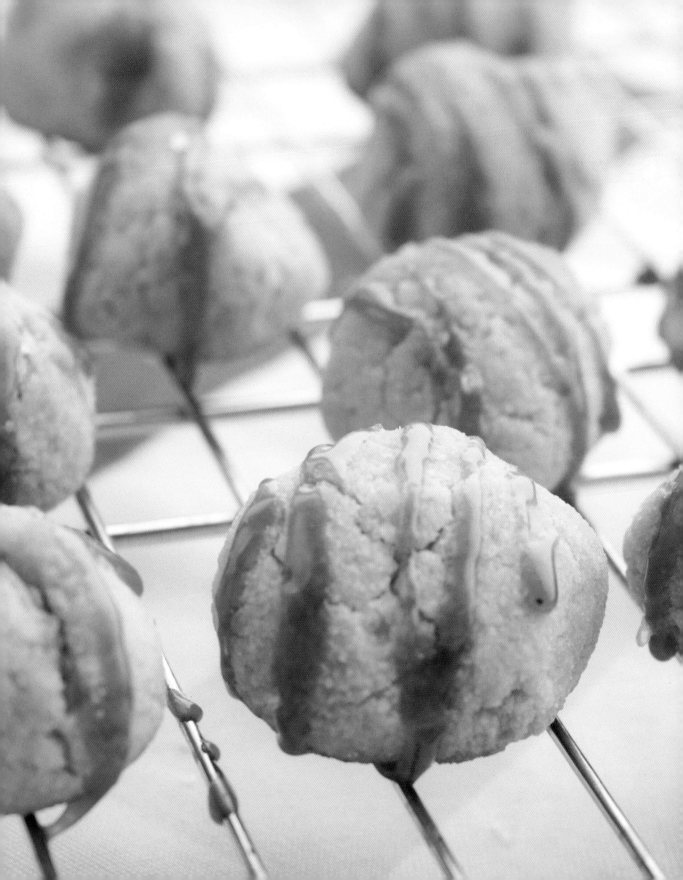

These **chewy, bite-size treats** combine the sweetness of coconut and maple syrup with sea salt for a mouthful of flavor.

Caramel Coconut
Macaroons

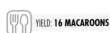 YIELD: **16 MACAROONS**   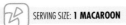 SERVING SIZE: **1 MACAROON**   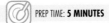 PREP TIME: **5 MINUTES**   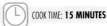 COOK TIME: **15 MINUTES**

INGREDIENTS

1½ cups unsweetened shredded coconut

2 TB. coconut oil

2 TB. coconut flour

1 TB. vanilla extract

¼ cup maple syrup

¼ tsp. sea salt

¼ cup **Sea Salt Caramel Sauce**

SPECIAL TOOLS

 FOOD PROCESSOR

METHOD

1 Preheat the oven to 350°F (180°C). Line a baking sheet with parchment paper.

2 In a food processor, combine shredded coconut, coconut oil, coconut flour, vanilla extract, maple syrup, and sea salt. Process for 30 seconds or until ingredients are well combined and have the texture of wet sand.

3 Scoop batter onto the baking sheet in 1-tablespoon portions.

4 Bake for 10 minutes. Rotate the pan and bake for another 5 minutes or until golden brown.

5 Let cool on pan for 5 to 10 minutes before transferring to cooling rack. When completely cool, drizzle with Sea Salt Caramel Sauce.

Storage: Store in an airtight container for up to 1 week.

NUTRITION

Calories 59	Saturated Fat 4g	Cholesterol 0mg	Carbohydrate 5g	Sugar 4g
Total Fat 4g	Unsaturated Fat 0g	Sodium 39mg	Dietary Fiber 1g	Protein 1g

Hearty greens are at the core of this juice, but the **lemon, apple, and ginger** provide a tart and spicy lift.

Green Lemonade

 YIELD: **16 OUNCES (450ML)**   SERVING SIZE: **8 OUNCES (225ML)**   PREP TIME: **35 MINUTES**   COOK TIME: **NONE**

INGREDIENTS

1 cup kale (1 large leaf)

1 cup romaine lettuce (2 large leaves)

1 cup spinach

3 cups Granny Smith apple, cored and roughly chopped (1½ large apples)

½ medium lemon, rind removed

1 (1-inch; 2.5cm) piece fresh ginger, peeled

3 cups cucumber, peeled (1 medium cucumber)

METHOD

1 Place kale, romaine lettuce, and spinach in a large bowl. Cover greens with water and soak for 30 minutes. (This will allow the juicer to extract the maximum juice from the leaves.)

2 One at a time, put kale, romaine, spinach, apple, lemon, ginger, and cucumber in the juicer. Juice each ingredient and stir to combine.

Storage: Store in an airtight jar and keep refrigerated for up to 48 hours.

> Challenge yourself to eat three colors at every meal. The different colors of fruits and vegetables are reflective of the different types of compounds they contain. Dark leafy greens are rich in vitamins A, C, and K.

SPECIAL TOOLS

 JUICER

NUTRITION

| Calories 84 | Saturated Fat 0g | Cholesterol 0mg | Carbohydrate 20g | Sugar 10g |
| Total Fat 1g | Unsaturated Fat 0g | Sodium 31mg | Dietary Fiber 0g | Protein 3g |

The **light and refreshing flavors** of celery and cucumber are complemented with fresh mint and a hint of lime in this **verdant summer cooler**.

Cucumber Mint Refresher

 YIELD: **16 OUNCES (450ML)**   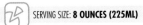 SERVING SIZE: **8 OUNCES (225ML)**   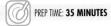 PREP TIME: **35 MINUTES**   COOK TIME: **NONE**

INGREDIENTS

2 cups spinach

1 cup fresh mint

3 cups cucumber, peeled
(1 medium cucumber)

1 small lime, rind removed

1 cup pineapple, rind removed
and roughly chopped

1 medium celery stalk

SPECIAL TOOLS

 JUICER

METHOD

1 Place spinach and mint in a large bowl. Cover with water and soak for 30 minutes. (This will allow the juicer to extract the maximum amount of juice from the leaves.)

2 One at a time, put spinach, mint, cucumber, lime, pineapple, and celery in the juicer. Juice each ingredient and stir to combine.

Storage: Store in an airtight jar and keep refrigerated for up to 48 hours.

NUTRITION

Calories **73**	Saturated Fat **0g**	Cholesterol **0mg**	Carbohydrate **17g**	Sugar **9g**
Total Fat **0g**	Unsaturated Fat **0g**	Sodium **47mg**	Dietary Fiber **0g**	Protein **3g**

Get your greens easily with this nutrient-packed beverage. Avocado adds the perfect creamy texture to this **citrusy green smoothie**.

Avocado Pineapple
Smoothie

 YIELD: **10 OUNCES (300ML)**   SERVING SIZE: **10 OUNCES (300ML)**   PREP TIME: **2 MINUTES**   COOK TIME: **NONE**

INGREDIENTS

1 cup kale, chopped and tightly packed

1 cup orange juice

½ cup pineapple, roughly chopped

¼ cup avocado, chopped

4–5 ice cubes

METHOD

1 In a blender, combine kale, orange juice, pineapple, avocado, and ice cubes.

2 Blend for 30 seconds or until smooth.

Storage: Smoothie is best enjoyed immediately.

SPECIAL TOOLS

 BLENDER

NUTRITION

Calories 218	Saturated Fat 1g	Cholesterol 0mg	Carbohydrate 34g	Sugar 18g
Total Fat 9g	Unsaturated Fat 10g	Sodium 34mg	Dietary Fiber 6g	Protein 5g

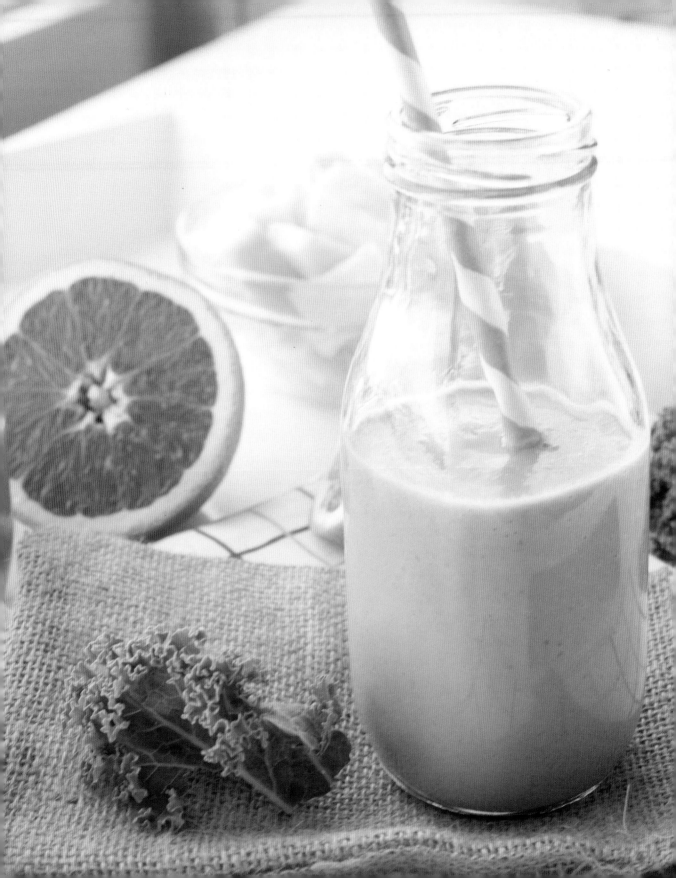

The **sweetness of carrots** and the **tart flavors of pineapple and lemon** come together in this refreshing juice, which features a **zesty ginger kick**.

Carrot Pineapple Juice

 YIELD: **16 OUNCES (450ML)**   SERVING SIZE: **8 OUNCES (225ML)**   PREP TIME: **10 MINUTES**   COOK TIME: **NONE**

INGREDIENTS

4–5 medium carrots, peeled

½ medium lemon, rind removed

1 cup pineapple, chopped

1 (1-in.; 2.5cm) piece fresh ginger, peeled

1 medium cucumber, peeled

SPECIAL TOOLS

 JUICER

METHOD

1 One at a time, put carrots, lemon, pineapple, ginger, and cucumber in the juicer.

2 Juice each ingredient and stir to combine.

Storage: Store in an airtight jar and keep refrigerated for up to 48 hours.

Serving Suggestion: This juice can be enjoyed first thing in the morning, as a nutritious complement to your breakfast, or as an afternoon pick-me-up.

Ginger contains anti-inflammatory compounds called gingerols that can help soothe the intestinal tract and relieve joint pain.

NUTRITION

| Calories 131 | Saturated Fat 0g | Cholesterol 0mg | Carbohydrate 32g | Sugar 17g |
| Total Fat 1g | Unsaturated Fat 0g | Sodium 109mg | Dietary Fiber 0g | Protein 3g |

The earthy flavor of beets is balanced with the sweetness of apple and carrots in this **nutrient-rich, vibrant, and colorful juice**.

Apple Beet Elixir

 YIELD: **16 OUNCES (450ML)**   SERVING SIZE: **8 OUNCES (225ML)**   PREP TIME: **10 MINUTES**   COOK TIME: **NONE**

INGREDIENTS

1 small beet, peeled and roughly chopped

4–5 medium carrots, peeled

1 (1-in.; 2.5cm) piece fresh ginger, peeled

1 lemon, rind removed

1 large apple, cored and roughly chopped

METHOD

1 One at a time, put beet, carrots, ginger, lemon, and apple in the juicer.

2 Juice each ingredient and stir to combine.

Storage: Store in an airtight jar and keep refrigerated for up to 48 hours.

The nitrates in beets dilate blood vessels and allow more oxygen and nutrients to reach working muscles in the body. This increases the efficiency of oxygen utilization for energy production during exercise.

SPECIAL TOOLS

 JUICER

NUTRITION

| Calories 156 | Saturated Fat 0g | Cholesterol 0mg | Carbohydrate 39g | Sugar 23g |
| Total Fat 1g | Unsaturated Fat 0g | Sodium 160mg | Dietary Fiber 0g | Protein 3g |

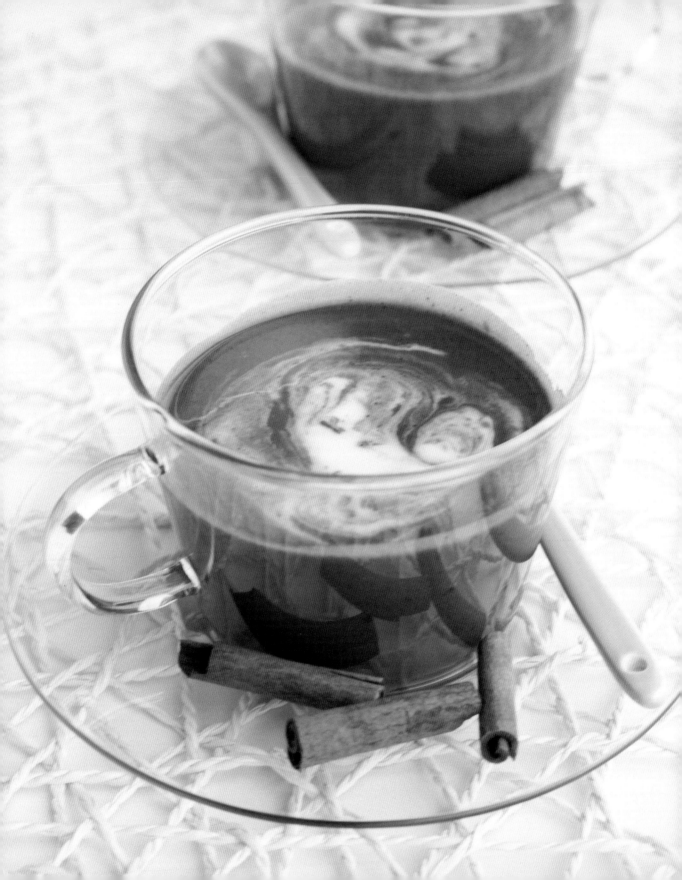

Enjoy a warm cup of hot "cocoa" on a cold day with this **dairy-free coconut milk** version featuring **rich carob powder** and **sweet maple syrup**.

Creamy Coconut Milk
Hot Cocoa

 YIELD: **2 CUPS**   SERVING SIZE: **1 CUP**   PREP TIME: **2 MINUTES**   COOK TIME: **5 MINUTES**

INGREDIENTS

2 cups light coconut milk

2 TB. carob powder

2 TB. maple syrup

1 tsp. vanilla extract

½ tsp. cinnamon

¼ cup water

METHOD

1 In a small saucepan over low heat, whisk together coconut milk, carob powder, maple syrup, vanilla extract, cinnamon, and water.

2 Heat for 5 minutes, stirring frequently, until contents are combined and warm.

Storage: Cocoa is best served immediately.

Serving Suggestion: Serve warm topped with a dollop of Coconut Whipped Cream.

NUTRITION

Calories 241	Saturated Fat 11g	Cholesterol 0mg	Carbohydrate 39g	Sugar 27g
Total Fat 12g	Unsaturated Fat 0g	Sodium 82mg	Dietary Fiber 9g	Protein 1g

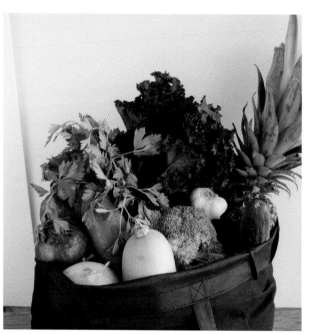

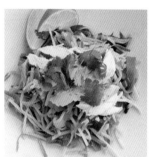

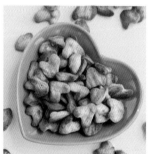

CHAPTER 9

Meal Plans

& Shopping Lists

Using Meal Plans
and Shopping Lists

The following pages include six weeks of meal plans, along with shopping lists, to guide you in considering what to eat during the weeks ahead.

About the Meals

Whether you are new to the AIP diet or are looking for some new recipes to spice up your meals, the meal plans for each week are structured to maximize your time and leftovers while still offering variety.

Breakfasts

Each week includes two different breakfast options. Breakfast items can all be made ahead of time.

Lunches

Lunches are either simple salads that can be prepped ahead of time or meals from a previous night's dinner.

Dinners

More complex dinner recipes are scheduled for the weekend, while easier recipes are suggested for weeknight meals.

About the Shopping Lists

Each plan is accompanied by a corresponding shopping list to make your life easier.

Quantities: Each shopping list includes the exact quantities of ingredients needed for all of the recipes within the week.

Inventory: Before you go shopping, take an inventory of your current fridge, freezer, and pantry and cross off items you already have to avoid overbuying.

Staples: Many of the weekly meal plans include staple recipes like Worcestershire Sauce and Seed-Free Curry Powder. If you already have these on hand, eliminate those ingredients from the shopping list.

Avoid Temptation

Avoid the temptation of foods that are not AIP-friendly by visiting the grocery store less frequently. Try shopping only once a week, and choose a day when you have time to peruse the supermarket shelves consciously and carefully.

Things to **Consider**

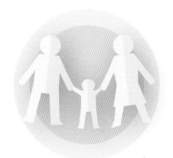

Family Size: Depending on how many individuals you cook for in your household, some of these recipes may stretch farther than what's listed. Take this opportunity to freeze leftovers for when you need a meal in a pinch.

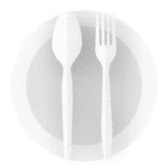

New Recipes vs. Leftovers: The meal plans are structured to make the most of leftovers. Note that recipes in **bold** need to be made from scratch.

Perfect Pairings: Many main course recipes are paired with side dish recipes to create a complete meal. These side dishes are simply suggestions, so feel free to mix and match different side dishes to the main courses as you begin to identify your favorite recipes.

Tools and Appliances: Each recipe lists any special tools needed to create the dish. Reference each recipe to ensure you have the necessary tools to make a dish before you begin your planning and shopping.

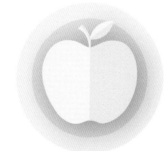

Fruit and Salads: If you require larger serving sizes than those suggested throughout the book, feel free to double the serving size, or add something simple to the meal like fresh fruit to your breakfast or a side salad with your dinner.

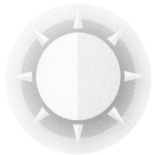

Practice and Have Fun! The more you practice, the easier planning becomes. The AIP diet is an opportunity for you to try new foods, build a list of your favorite go-to recipes, and involve your friends and family in your new way of cooking and eating.

Week 1 Meal Plan

	SUNDAY	MONDAY	TUESDAY
BREAKFAST	Crisp Ham Cups Root Vegetable Breakfast Hash	Key Lime No'gurt	Crisp Ham Cups Root Vegetable Breakfast Hash
LUNCH	Mediterranean Tuna Salad	Wild Mushroom and Meatball Stew	Mediterranean Tuna Salad
DINNER	Wild Mushroom and Meatball Stew	Herbed Baked Spaghetti Squash Tomato-Less Pasta Sauce	Middle Eastern Bison Burgers Sea Salt Kale Crisps

Shopping List

STAPLE RECIPES

Seed-Free Curry Powder

Worcestershire Sauce

PROTEINS

Deli ham (12 slices)	Ground bison (1 lb.; 450g)	Salmon filet, skin on (1 lb.; 450g)
Pancetta (¼ cup)	Ground turkey, dark meat (1 lb.; 450g)	
Ground pork (1 lb.; 450g)		

PRODUCE

Yellow onions (4)	Fresh rosemary (3 TB.)	Beet (1 small)	Fennel (½ bulb)
Red onion (1)	Fresh oregano (1 TB.)	Spaghetti squash (1 medium)	Mushrooms (8 cups)
Shallot (1)	Fresh ginger (2 TB.)	Avocados (3)	Kale (12 cups; about 10 leaves)
Garlic (17 cloves)	Fresh basil (¼ cup)	Cucumber (½)	Butter lettuce (2 heads; about 16 large leaves)
Green onions (6)	Purple sweet potato (1)	Cauliflower (1 head)	Pineapple (2 cups)
Parsley (1 cup)	Rutabaga (1)	Celery (2 stalks)	
Fresh thyme (¼ cup)	Carrots (5)	Lime (1)	
Chives (½ tsp.)	Parsnip (1)	Lemon (1)	

WEDNESDAY	THURSDAY	FRIDAY	SATURDAY
Key Lime No'gurt	Crisp Ham Cups Root Vegetable Breakfast Hash	Key Lime No'gurt	Crisp Ham Cups Root Vegetable Breakfast Hash
Middle Eastern Bison Burgers Sea Salt Kale Crisps	Mediterranean Tuna Salad	Wild Mushroom and Meatball Stew	Pineapple Teriyaki Salmon Cauliflower Fried Rice
Herbed Baked Spaghetti Squash Tomato-Less Pasta Sauce	Asian Turkey Lettuce Wraps	Pineapple Teriyaki Salmon Cauliflower Fried Rice	Asian Turkey Lettuce Wraps

PANTRY ITEMS

Olive oil (1 cup)	Lemon juice (¼ cup)
Coconut oil (1 TB.)	Beef broth (4 cups)
Ghee (4 TB.)	Vegetable broth (2 cups)
Apple cider vinegar (1 cup)	Sweet potato purée (2 TB.)
Balsamic vinegar (1 TB.)	Water chestnuts (1 [113g] can)
Coconut aminos (¾ cup)	Arrowroot powder (2 TB.)
Fish sauce (3 TB.)	Albacore tuna (4 [6-oz; 170g] cans)
Maple syrup (½ cup)	Artichoke hearts (1 [14-oz; 395g] can)
Honey (3 TB.)	Green olives (¾ cup)
Molasses (1 TB.)	
Lime juice (3 TB.)	

SPICES

Sea salt (3⅛ tsp.)	Dried turmeric (1½ tsp.)
Dried basil (2 tsp.)	Dried cilantro (1 tsp.)
Dried thyme (1 tsp.)	Dried dill weed (½ tsp.)
Dried oregano (2 tsp.)	Ground cinnamon (½ tsp.)
Onion powder (2 tsp.)	Ground ginger (½ tsp.)
Garlic powder (1¾ tsp.)	Ground cloves (¾ tsp.)

OTHER

Pitted prunes (about 10)

Bacon fat (2 TB.)

Week 2 Meal Plan

	SUNDAY	MONDAY	TUESDAY
BREAKFAST	Apple Cinnamon Hearts Cereal	Rosemary and Thyme Sausage Patties Root Vegetable Breakfast Hash	Apple Cinnamon Hearts Cereal
LUNCH	Avocado Chicken Salad	Triple-Berry Barbecue Ribs Honey Vinegar Tri-Colored Slaw	Roasted Butternut Squash and Sage Soup Celeriac Apple Currant Slaw
DINNER	Triple-Berry Barbecue Ribs Honey Vinegar Tri-Colored Slaw	Roasted Butternut Squash and Sage Soup Celeriac Apple Currant Slaw	Greek-Style Roast Chicken

Shopping List

STAPLE RECIPES

Triple-Berry Barbecue Sauce

Worcestershire Sauce

PROTEINS

Ground pork (1 lb.; 450g)	Whole roasting chicken, without giblets (4½ lb.; 2.1kg)	Boneless, skinless chicken breast (1lb.; 450g)
Lamb stew meat (1 lb.; 450g)	Rack ribs (3 lbs.; 1.5kg)	

PRODUCE

Yellow onions (3)	Chives (½ tsp.)	Carrots (5)	Jicama (1)
Red onions (2)	Fresh basil (2 TB.)	Parsnip (1)	Red cabbage (3 cups)
Green onions (6)	Cilantro (¾ cup)	Granny Smith apples (3)	Green cabbage (3 cups)
Shallots (2)	Fresh ginger (1 tsp.)	Butternut squash (1 medium)	Avocados (2)
Garlic (23 cloves)	Sweet potatoes (2 medium)	Limes (1½)	Mango (1)
Fresh rosemary (2 tsp.)	Purple sweet potato (1)	Lemons (5)	Strawberries (⅓ cup)
Fresh thyme (1 TB. + 2 tsp.)	Celery root (4 cups)	Mixed greens (4 cups)	Blueberries (⅓ cup)
Fresh sage (¼ cup)	Rutabaga (1)	Cucumbers (3½)	Cherries, frozen (⅓ cup)

WEDNESDAY	THURSDAY	FRIDAY	SATURDAY
Rosemary and Thyme Sausage Patties Root Vegetable Breakfast Hash	Apple Cinnamon Hearts Cereal	Rosemary and Thyme Sausage Patties Root Vegetable Breakfast Hash	Apple Cinnamon Hearts Cereal
Caribbean Chicken Salad Cilantro Lime Vinaigrette	Avocado Chicken Salad	Roasted Butternut Squash and Sage Soup Celeriac Apple Currant Slaw	Burgundy Lamb Kabobs Asian Cucumber Salad
Burgundy Lamb Kabobs Asian Cucumber Salad	Greek-Style Roast Chicken	Burgundy Lamb Kabobs Asian Cucumber Salad	Caribbean Chicken Salad Cilantro Lime Vinaigrette

PANTRY ITEMS

Olive oil (1 cup + 5 TB.)

Coconut oil (¼ cup)

Ghee (2 TB.)

White wine vinegar (1 TB.)

Sherry vinegar (1 TB.)

Apple cider vinegar (¾ cup)

Coconut aminos (2 TB.)

Fish sauce (2 TB.)

Honey (¼ cup + 2 TB.)

Maple syrup (½ cup + 1 TB.)

Molasses (3 TB.)

Lime juice (¼ cup)

Bone Broth or chicken broth (4½ cups)

Beef broth (1 cup)

Light coconut milk (1 cup)

Coconut flour (½ cup)

Arrowroot powder (½ cup)

SPICES

Sea salt (5½ tsp.)

Ground cinnamon (1 tsp.)

Dried parsley (1½ TB.)

Dried oregano (2 TB.)

Garlic powder (½ tsp.)

Onion powder (¾ tsp.)

Ground cloves (¼ tsp.)

Vanilla extract (2 tsp.)

OTHER

Bacon fat (¼ cup)

Unsweetened applesauce (1 cup)

Orange juice (¼ cup)

Currants (½ cup)

Dried cranberries (¼ cup)

Unsweetened shredded coconut (¼ cup)

Red wine (1 cup)

Week 3 Meal Plan

	SUNDAY	MONDAY	TUESDAY
BREAKFAST	Carrot Cake Waffles	Sweet & Spicy Gra'no'la	Carrot Cake Waffles
LUNCH	Tuscan Sausage and Kale Soup Hasselback Sweet Potatoes	Grilled Chicken Cobb Salad Greek Red Wine Vinaigrette	Tuscan Sausage and Kale Soup Hasselback Sweet Potatoes
DINNER	Blackened Chicken Breast Pad Thai Noodles	Chimichurri Skirt Steak Hasselback Sweet Potatoes	Orange Pulled Pork Carnitas Pan-Seared Brussels Sprouts with Bacon

Shopping List

STAPLE RECIPES

Seed-Free Curry Powder

PROTEINS

Skirt steak (1 lb.; 450g)

Pork sausage (½ lb.; 225g)

Bacon (10 slices)

Boneless pork shoulder (3½ lb.; 1.6kg)

Boneless pork tenderloin (1 lb.; 450g)

Boneless, skinless chicken breast (2 lb.; 900g)

PRODUCE

Yellow onion (1)

White onion (1)

Red onion (1)

Shallot (½)

Green onions (6)

Garlic (21 cloves)

Fresh rosemary (1 TB.)

Fresh sage (1 TB.)

Parsley (2½ cups)

Cilantro (¼ cup)

Sweet potatoes (4 medium)

Carrots (2 lb.; 900g)

Butternut squash (1 cup)

Plantains, ripe or green (3 cups)

Avocado (1)

Cucumber (2 cups)

Zucchini (1)

Brussels sprouts (1 lb.; 450g)

Broccoli slaw (3 cups)

Kale (2 cups)

Romaine lettuce (8 cups)

Arugula (2 cups)

Lime (1)

Orange (1)

WEDNESDAY	THURSDAY	FRIDAY	SATURDAY
Sweet & Spicy Gra'no'la	Carrot Cake Waffles	Sweet & Spicy Gra'no'la	Carrot Cake Waffles
Blackened Chicken Breast Pad Thai Noodles	Grilled Chicken Cobb Salad Greek Red Wine Vinaigrette	Pork Tenderloin with Roasted Carrot Romesco	Tuscan Sausage and Kale Soup Hasselback Sweet Potatoes
Chimichurri Skirt Steak Hasselback Sweet Potatoes	**Pork Tenderloin with Roasted Carrot Romesco**	Orange Pulled Pork Carnitas Pan-Seared Brussels Sprouts with Bacon	Orange Pulled Pork Carnitas Pan-Seared Brussels Sprouts with Bacon

PANTRY ITEMS

Olive oil (1 cup + 2 TB.)

Coconut oil (¼ cup + 3 TB.)

Ghee (3 TB.)

Apple cider vinegar (2 TB.)

Red wine vinegar (¼ cup)

Sherry vinegar (3 TB.)

Lime juice (¼ cup)

Lemon juice (¼ cup + 1 TB.)

Coconut aminos (2 TB.)

Fish sauce (¼ cup)

Maple syrup (¼ cup)

Coconut butter (1 TB.)

Chicken broth (4 cups)

Light coconut milk (½ cup)

Pumpkin purée (½ cup)

Sweet potato purée (¼ cup)

Arrowroot powder (½ cup)

Baking soda (2 tsp.)

SPICES

Sea salt (3 tsp.)

Cinnamon (2 tsp.)

Cream of tartar (1 tsp.)

Ground ginger (1 tsp.)

Bay leaves (2)

Dried oregano (4 TB. + ½ tsp.)

Dried thyme (1½ tsp.)

Garlic powder (3 tsp.)

Onion powder (1½ tsp.)

Dried turmeric (1½ tsp.)

Dried cilantro (1 tsp.)

Dried basil (1 tsp.)

Dried dill weed (½ tsp.)

Ground cloves (¼ tsp.)

OTHER

Unsweetened banana chips (½ cup)

Unsweetened dried mango (½ cup)

Raisins (½ cup)

Unsweetened coconut flakes (2 cups)

Coconut sugar (1½ tsp.)

Week 4 Meal Plan

	SUNDAY	MONDAY	TUESDAY
BREAKFAST	Okonomiyaki	Zesty Lemon No'gurt	Okonomiyaki
LUNCH	Parsnip Seafood Chowder	Sunday Slow Cooker Pot Roast Parsnip Purée	Homestyle Meatloaf Muffins Cranberry Orange Relish
DINNER	Sunday Slow Cooker Pot Roast Parsnip Purée	Homestyle Meatloaf Muffins Cranberry Orange Relish	Apple Cider Pork Chops Roasted Balsamic Green Beans

Shopping List

STAPLE RECIPES

Worcestershire Sauce

PROTEINS

Bacon (6 slices)

Bone-in pork chops (1 lb.; 450g)

Flank steak (1 lb.; 450g)

Boneless chuck roast
(3 lb.; 1.5kg)

Ground beef (1 lb.; 450g)

Shrimp, peeled and deveined
(½ lb.; 225g)

Bay scallops (½ lb.; 225g)

Monkfish (or other mild white fish)
(½ lb.; 225g)

Crab meat (½ lb.; 225g)

PRODUCE

Yellow onions (4)

Shallots (2 cups)

Garlic (21 cloves)

Green onions (6)

Leeks (2)

Fresh thyme (3 TB. + 1 tsp.)

Fresh ginger (1 TB. + 1 tsp.)

Parsley (1 cup)

Carrots (2 medium)

Mint (1 TB.)

Sweet potatoes (3 large)

Parsnips (9–12)

Celery (4 stalks)

Zucchini (1)

Green cabbage (3 cups)

Cauliflower (2 medium heads)

Broccoli (1 small head)

Green beans (1 lb.; 450g)

Avocados (2)

Apples (2 large)

Oranges (2)

Grapefruit (1)

Pomegranate (1)

Lemon (1)

Whole cranberries (4 cups)

WEDNESDAY	THURSDAY	FRIDAY	SATURDAY
Zesty Lemon No'gurt	Okonomiyaki	Zesty Lemon No'gurt	Okonomiyaki
Sunday Slow Cooker Pot Roast Parsnip Purée	Broccoli Beef Stir-Fry Cauliflower Fried Rice	Parsnip Seafood Chowder	Cauliflower Leek Soup Citrus Mint Salad
Broccoli Beef Stir-Fry Cauliflower Fried Rice	Apple Cider Pork Chops Roasted Balsamic Green Beans	**Cauliflower Leek Soup Citrus Mint Salad**	Parsnip Seafood Chowder

PANTRY ITEMS

Olive oil (½ cup)

Coconut oil (2 TB.)

Ghee (½ cup)

Balsamic vinegar (4 tsp.)

White wine vinegar (1 tsp.)

Apple cider vinegar (½ cup)

Coconut aminos (½ cup + 1 TB.)

Fish sauce (¼ cup)

Lemon juice (3 TB. + 1 tsp.)

Lime juice (3 TB.)

Maple syrup (1⅓ cup + 2 TB.)

Honey (3 TB. + 1 tsp.)

Molasses (1 TB.)

Chicken broth (5 cups)

Vegetable broth (½ cup)

Beef broth (2 cups)

Clam juice (1 cup)

Unsweetened applesauce (⅓ cup)

Light coconut milk (2½ [13.5-oz; 400ml] cans)

Coconut flour (⅓ cup + 2 TB.)

Arrowroot powder (1 tsp.)

Tapioca starch (1 TB. + 1 tsp.)

SPICES

Sea salt (2¾ tsp.)

Smoked sea salt (¼ tsp.)

Bay leaf (1)

Marjoram (1 tsp.)

Dried oregano (1 tsp.)

Onion powder (2 tsp.)

Garlic powder (2 tsp.)

Powdered turmeric (1½ tsp.)

Dried cilantro (1 tsp.)

Dried basil (2 tsp.)

Dried dill (½ tsp.)

Cinnamon (½ tsp.)

Ground ginger (1½ tsp.)

Ground cloves (2¾ tsp.)

OTHER

Bacon fat (1 TB.)

Golden raisins (½ cup)

Orange juice (1 cup)

100% apple juice (1½ cup)

Week 5 Meal Plan

	SUNDAY	MONDAY	TUESDAY
BREAKFAST	Apple Cinnamon No-Oat Oatmeal	Carrot Cake Waffles	Apple Cinnamon No-Oat Oatmeal
LUNCH	Shaved Broccoli and Cauliflower Slaw	Bacon-Wrapped Scallops Roasted Broccolini with White Wine Mushrooms	Crispy Chicken Strips with Mango Honey Sauce Rosemary Sweet Potato Chips
DINNER	Bacon-Wrapped Scallops Roasted Broccolini with White Wine Mushrooms	Crispy Chicken Strips with Mango Honey Sauce Rosemary Sweet Potato Chips	Honey Ginger Glazed Salmon Rutabaga Purée

Shopping List

STAPLE RECIPES

None

PROTEINS

Large sea scallops (1 lb.; 450g)

Bacon (12 slices)

Pancetta (2 oz.; 55g)

Boneless, skinless chicken breast (1 lb.; 450g)

Salmon filet, skin on (1 lb.; 450g)

PRODUCE

Shallot (1 medium)

Green onions (5)

Garlic (7 cloves)

Cilantro (2 TB.)

Fresh basil (2 cups)

Fresh ginger (1 TB.)

Parsley (1 cup)

Fresh rosemary (2 TB.)

Sweet potatoes (2 medium)

Rutabaga (1)

Butternut squash (½)

Carrots (6)

Broccoli (1 large head)

Broccolini (2 bunches)

Cauliflower (2 heads)

Zucchini (8 medium)

Baby bella mushrooms (8 oz.; 225g)

Kale (1 large bunch)

Avocado (1)

Plantains (2)

Lime (1)

Lemon (1)

Orange (1)

Mango (1)

WEDNESDAY	THURSDAY	FRIDAY	SATURDAY
Carrot Cake Waffles	Apple Cinnamon No-Oat Oatmeal	Carrot Cake Waffles	Apple Cinnamon No-Oat Oatmeal
Shaved Broccoli and Cauliflower Slaw	**Classic Kale Salad**	Classic Kale Salad	Crispy Chicken Strips with Mango Honey Sauce Rosemary Sweet Potato Chips
Honey Ginger Glazed Salmon Rutabaga Purée	**Garlic Pesto Zucchini Pasta**	Garlic Pesto Zucchini Pasta	Shaved Broccoli and Cauliflower Slaw

PANTRY ITEMS		SPICES	
Olive oil (1¾ cup + 1 TB.)	Coconut aminos (¼ cup)	Sea salt (1½ tsp.)	Dried basil (1 tsp.)
Coconut oil (¼ cup)	Light coconut milk (4½ cups)	Smoked sea salt (¼ tsp.)	Powdered turmeric (1½ tsp.)
Ghee (2 TB.)	Pumpkin purée (½ cup)	Garlic powder (2¼ tsp.)	Ground cloves (½ tsp.)
Apple cider vinegar (1 TB. + 1 tsp.)	Unsweetened applesauce (1 cup)	Onion powder (2 tsp.)	Cinnamon (2½ tsp.)
Sherry vinegar (1 TB.)	Maple syrup (¼ cup)	Dried oregano (1⅛ tsp.)	Ground ginger (1 tsp.)
Red wine vinegar (2 TB.)	Honey (¼ cup + 2 TB.)	Dried thyme (⅛ tsp.)	Cream of tartar (1 tsp.)
Lime juice (1 TB.)	Arrowroot powder (½ cup + 2 TB.)	Dried dill (½ tsp.)	Vanilla extract (1 tsp.)
Lemon juice (1 cup)	Coconut flour (2 TB.)	Dried cilantro (1 tsp.)	
	Baking soda (2 tsp.)		

OTHER			
Bacon fat (1 TB.)	Pineapple juice (½ cup)	Unsweetened shredded coconut (1½ cup)	Dried cranberries (⅓ cup)
White wine (¼ cup)	Orange juice (¼ cup)	Raisins (2½ cups)	Apricot preserves (¼ cup)

Week 6 Meal Plan

	SUNDAY	MONDAY	TUESDAY
BREAKFAST	Sweet & Spicy Gra'no'la	Apple Cinnamon Hearts Cereal	Sweet & Spicy Gra'no'la
LUNCH	Spring Asparagus and Broccoli Soup	Spring Asparagus and Broccoli Soup	Mexican Carnitas Broth Bowl
DINNER	Mexican Carnitas Broth Bowl	Mexican Carnitas Broth Bowl	Lemon-Stuffed Sea Bass Garlic Caper Roasted Cauliflower

Shopping List

STAPLE RECIPES	PROTEINS		
None	Shrimp, peeled and deveined (1 lb.; 450g)	Salmon fillet, skin on (1 lb.; 450g)	Boneless pork shoulder (3½ lb.; 1.6kg)
	Whole sea bass, cleaned (about 2 lb.; 1 kg)	Duck breast, skin on (1 lb.; 450g))	Pancetta (2 oz.; 55g)

PRODUCE

Red onion (1)	Fresh thyme (4 TB. + ½ tsp.)	Broccoli (1 small head)
Shallot (1 large)	Rosemary (5 sprigs)	Jicama (1 small)
Garlic (17 cloves)	Butternut squash (1 medium)	Avocados (2)
White onion (1)	Chayote squash (1 medium)	Lemon (2)
Green onions (4)	Carrots (4–5)	Limes (4)
Leeks (2 large)	Arugula (2 cups)	Mango (1)
Parsley (½ cup)	Cauliflower (1 head)	Orange (1)
Cilantro (¾ cup)	Asparagus (1 lb.; 450g)	

WEDNESDAY	THURSDAY	FRIDAY	SATURDAY
Apple Cinnamon Hearts Cereal	Sweet & Spicy Gra'no'la	Apple Cinnamon Hearts Cereal	Sweet & Spicy Gra'no'la
Citrus Shrimp Ceviche	Lemon-Stuffed Sea Bass Garlic Caper Roasted Cauliflower	Citrus Shrimp Ceviche	Spring Asparagus and Broccoli Soup
Roast Duck with Shallots, Figs, and Honey Cinnamon Hasselback Sweet Potatoes	Maple Balsamic Glazed Salmon Savory Baked Butternut Squash	Roast Duck with Shallots, Figs, and Honey Cinnamon Hasselback Sweet Potatoes	Maple Balsamic Glazed Salmon Savory Baked Butternut Squash

PANTRY ITEMS

Olive oil (¾ cup + 1 TB.)	Molasses (1 TB.)
Coconut oil (¼ cup + 2 TB.)	Honey (2 TB.)
Coconut butter (1 TB.)	Light coconut milk (1 cup)
Apple cider vinegar (¼ cup)	Coconut flour (½ cup)
Balsamic vinegar (¼ cup)	Arrowroot powder (½ cup)
Lemon juice (¼ cup + 2 TB.)	
Lime juice (1 cup)	
Vegetable broth (2½ cups)	
Chicken broth (4 cups)	
Capers (2 TB.)	
Maple syrup (½ cup)	
Unsweetened applesauce (1 cup)	

SPICES

Sea salt (2½ tsp.)	Dried cilantro (1 tsp.)
Dried oregano (1 TB. + 1 tsp.)	Dried basil (1 tsp.)
Cinnamon (3 tsp.)	Dried dill (½ tsp.)
Onion powder (1½ tsp.)	Ground ginger (½ tsp.)
Garlic powder (1½ tsp.)	Ground cloves (¼ tsp.)
Powdered turmeric (1½ tsp.)	Vanilla extract (2 tsp.)

OTHER

Unsweetened coconut flakes (2 cups)	Unsweetened banana chips (½ cup)
Coconut sugar (½ tsp.)	Bacon fat (2 TB.)
Dried figs (1 cup)	Dry white wine (½ cup)
	Red wine (½ cup + 1 tsp.)

Glossary

arrowroot   A starch extracted from the roots of the arrowroot plant.

artichoke heart   The center of the artichoke flower, often sold canned or frozen.

arugula   A spicy, peppery green that has a sharp, distinctive flavor.

bake   To cook in a dry oven.

baking powder   A dry ingredient used to increase volume and lighten or leaven baked goods.

balsamic vinegar   A heavy, dark, sweet vinegar produced primarily in Italy from a specific type of grape and aged in wood barrels.

basil   A flavorful, almost sweet, resinous herb delicious with tomatoes and used in many Italian- and Mediterranean-style dishes.

baste   To keep foods moist during cooking by applying a liquid.

beat   To quickly mix substances.

blanch   To place a food in boiling water for about a minute to partially cook and then douse with cool water to halt the cooking.

blend   To completely mix something, usually with a blender or food processor; slower than beating.

boil   To heat a liquid to the point water turns into steam, causing the liquid to bubble. Also to cook food in boiling water.

bok choy   A member of the cabbage family with thick stems, crisp texture, and fresh flavor. It's perfect for stir-frying.

braise   To cook with the introduction of a liquid, usually over a period of time.

broccolini   A hybrid of broccoli and kale with slender stalks and small florets.

broil   To cook in a dry oven under the overhead high-heat element.

broth   See stock.

brown   To cook in a skillet, turning, until the food's surface is seared and brown in color.

butternut squash   A bell-shaped winter squash with sweet orange-yellow flesh.

caper   The flavorful bud of a Mediterranean plant that is preserved in salt or vinegar.

caramelize   To cook vegetables or meat in butter or oil over low heat until they soften, sweeten, and develop a caramel color. Also to cook sugar over low heat until it develops a sweet caramel flavor.

carob   The flesh of tropical tree pods that are dried, baked, and powdered for use in baking. The flavor is similar to chocolate.

celeriac   A turnip-rooted celery variety with a knobby exterior and mild, crunchy flesh.

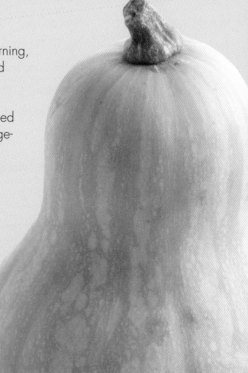

ceviche A seafood dish marinated for hours in lemon or lime juice, tomato, onion, and cilantro. The acidic citrus juice "cooks" the seafood.

chayote squash A gourd with a pear-like shape, pale lime green color, sweet flavor, and crispy texture.

chiffonade A chopping technique that involves shredding leafy vegetables into thin, ribbon-like pieces.

chive An herb that grows in bunches of long leaves and offers a light onion flavor.

chop To cut into pieces, usually qualified such as "coarsely chopped" or with a size measurement such as "chopped into ½-inch (1.25cm) pieces." "Finely chopped" is much closer to mince.

chutney A thick condiment often served with Indian curries made with fruits and/or vegetables with vinegar, sugar, and spices.

cider vinegar A vinegar produced from apple cider, popular in North America.

cilantro A member of the parsley family often used in Mexican dishes. The seed is called coriander in North America; elsewhere, the plant is called coriander.

cinnamon A rich, aromatic spice commonly used in baking or desserts.

clam juice The liquid strained from freshly shucked clams. It has a briny fresh fish taste that is used in many seafood dishes.

clove A sweet, strong, almost wintergreen-flavor spice used in baking.

coconut aminos A soy-free seasoning (similar in flavor to soy sauce) that is made by fermenting coconut tree sap.

coconut butter A thick and smooth butter made from the flesh of the coconut. It is thicker and richer than coconut oil.

coconut flour A soft dense flour derived from dried, ground coconut meat.

coconut milk A milk made from one part shredded coconut and one part water. Coconut milk comes in full-fat and light varieties.

coconut oil An oil extracted from the meat of the coconut fruit.

coconut sugar A sugar produced from the liquid sap of cut flower buds of the coconut palm tree.

Coconut products are versatile and often used in AIP cooking.

count In terms of seafood or other foods that come in small sizes, the number of the item that compose 1 pound (450g).

cremini mushroom A brown, richly flavored mushroom. The larger, fully grown version is the portobello.

curry powder A blend of rich and flavorful spices such as hot pepper, nutmeg, cumin, cinnamon, pepper, and turmeric.

dash A few drops, usually of a liquid, released by a quick shake.

dates A sweet dried fruit with a large inedible pit.

deglaze To scrape up bits of meat and seasonings left in a pan after cooking, usually by adding a liquid such as wine or broth, to create a flavorful stock.

dehydrator An appliance that circulates warm air around food to encourage the evaporation of its water content.

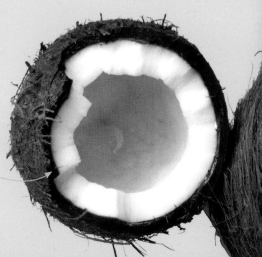

devein To remove the dark vein from the back of a large shrimp with a sharp knife.

dice To cut into small cubes about ¼-inch (.5cm) square.

dill A herb perfect for eggs, salmon, cheese dishes, and vegetables.

dredge To coat a piece of food on all sides with a dry substance such as flour or cornmeal.

emulsion A combination of liquid ingredients carefully and quickly beaten together to create a thick liquid, such as a fat or oil with water.

endive A green that resembles a small, elongated, tightly packed head of romaine lettuce. The thick, crunchy leaves can be broken off and used with dips and spreads.

extra-virgin olive oil See olive oil.

extract A concentrated flavoring derived from foods or plants through evaporation or distillation that imparts a powerful flavor without altering the volume or texture of a dish.

fennel In seed form, a fragrant, licorice-tasting herb. The bulbs have a mild flavor and a celery-like crunch.

figs A small, soft, pear-shaped fruit with a sweet, seedy flesh that can be eaten fresh or dried.

fish sauce A Thai and Vietnamese sauce known for its savory, sweet, and umami flavors that is extracted from fermented anchovies.

fold To combine a dense and a light mixture with a gentle move from the middle of the bowl outward to preserve the mixture's airy nature.

fry See sauté.

garlic A pungent and flavorful member of the onion family. A garlic bulb contains multiple cloves; each clove, when chopped, yields about 1 teaspoon garlic.

gelatin A substance derived from the collagen of animal by-products (skin, tendons, ligaments, and bones) that is commonly used in the production of jellies.

ghee A clarified butter made by heating butter to separate and remove the milk solids.

ginger A flavorful root available fresh or dried and ground that adds a pungent, sweet, and spicy quality to a dish.

golden raisin A raisin made from a white grape.

hearts of palm Firm, elongated, off-white cylinders from the inside of a palm tree stem tip.

horseradish A sharp, spicy root that can be grated and prepared as a condiment.

infusion A liquid in which flavorful ingredients such as herbs have been steeped to extract their flavor into the liquid.

Italian seasoning A blend of dried herbs, including basil, oregano, rosemary, and thyme.

jicama A large, round vegetable that's juicy, crunchy, and sweet. If you can't find jicama, substitute sliced water chestnuts.

julienne A French word meaning "to slice into very thin pieces."

kalamata olive Traditionally from Greece, a medium-small, long black olive with a rich, smoky flavor.

Key lime A very small lime grown primarily in Florida known for its tart taste.

kosher salt A coarse-grained salt made without additives or iodine.

leeks A long cylindrical vegetable resembling an oversized scallion with a sweet onion flavor.

marinate To soak a food in a seasoned sauce to impart flavor and make tender, as with meat.

marjoram A sweet herb similar to oregano, popular in Greek, Spanish, and Italian dishes.

mesclun Mixed salad greens such as lettuce, arugula, cress, and endive.

mince To cut into very small pieces, smaller than diced, about $1/8$ inch (3mm) or smaller.

monkfish A bottom-dwelling anglerfish with a white meaty texture and mild taste.

olive The green or black fruit of the olive tree.

olive oil A fragrant liquid produced by crushing or pressing olives. Extra-virgin olive oil, the most flavorful and highest quality, is produced from the olives' first pressing; oil is also produced from later pressings.

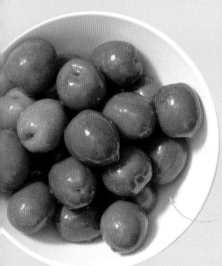

Olives make great snacks.

oregano A fragrant, slightly astringent herb used often in Greek, Spanish, and Italian dishes.

oxidation The gradual browning of a fruit or vegetable from exposure to air. Minimize oxidation by rubbing cut surfaces with lemon juice.

pancetta A salt-cured Italian bacon made from pork belly.

parboil To partially cook in boiling water or broth.

parsley A fresh-tasting green leafy herb, often used as a garnish.

parsnip A root vegetable that closely resembles a carrot, but with a white color and mild sweet flavor.

paté A mixture of cooked ground meat and fat minced together into a spreadable paste.

pesto A thick spread or sauce made with pine nuts, fresh basil, garlic, olive oil, and Parmesan cheese.

pinch An unscientific measurement for the amount of an ingredient you can hold between your finger and thumb.

poach To cook a food in simmering liquid such as water, wine, or broth.

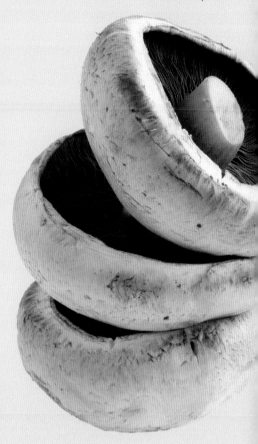

portobello mushroom A large, brown, chewy, flavorful mushroom.

preheat To turn on an oven, broiler, or other cooking appliance early so it will be hot when the dish is ready to be cooked.

prosciutto A dry-cured ham that is typically very thinly sliced.

purée To reduce a food to a thick, creamy texture, typically using a blender or food processor.

purple sweet potato A variety of sweet potato with a deep purple skin and vibrant purple flesh.

reduce   To boil or simmer a broth or sauce to remove some of the water content and yield a more concentrated flavor.

reserve   To hold a specified ingredient for use later in a recipe.

roast   To cook food uncovered in an oven, usually without additional liquid.

rosemary   A pungent, sweet herb used with chicken, pork, fish, and especially lamb.

rutabaga   A root vegetable with yellow flesh and a flavor similar to a turnip.

sage   An herb with a slightly musty, fruity, lemon-rind scent and earthy flavor.

sauté   To pan-cook over lower heat than what's used for frying.

scallops   Marine bivalve mollusks. Scallops come in a variety of sizes, including large sea scallops and small bay scallops.

sear   To quickly brown the exterior of a food, especially meat, over high heat.

shallot   A member of the onion family that grows in a bulb. Similar to garlic, but with a milder onion flavor.

shellfish   A broad range of seafood, including clams, mussels, oysters, crabs, shrimp, and lobster.

shiitake mushroom   A large, dark brown mushroom with a hearty, meaty flavor.

simmer   To boil gently so the liquid barely bubbles.

skillet (also frying pan)   A flat-bottomed metal pan with a handle designed to cook food on a stovetop.

skim   To remove fat or other material from the top of liquid.

smoked sea salt   A sea salt that has been naturally smoked over wood fires and gives a smoky aroma and flavor to food.

spaghetti squash   A winter squash with a bright yellow shell and a sweet flesh that, when cooked, resembles the texture and appearance of spaghetti noodles.

spiralized   A method of cutting vegetables using a spiralizer which carves long, thin, noodle-like pieces from vegetables.

steam   To suspend a food over boiling water and allow the heat of the steam to cook the food.

steep   To set something a liquid, as in steeping tea in hot water.

stew   To slowly cook pieces of food submerged in a liquid. Also a dish prepared using this method.

stir-fry   To cook small pieces of food in a wok or skillet over high heat, moving and turning the food quickly to cook all sides.

stock   A flavorful broth made by cooking meats and/or vegetables with seasonings until the liquid absorbs these flavors. The stock is strained, and the solids are discarded. Stock can be eaten alone or used as a base for soups, stews, etc.

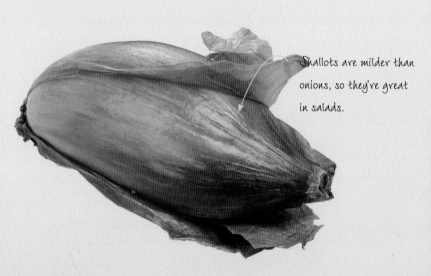

Shallots are milder than onions, so they're great in salads.

tapioca A starchy white flour extracted from the cassava plant.

tarragon A sweet, rich-smelling herb perfect with vegetables, seafood, chicken, and pork.

tartar sauce A mayonnaise-based sauce often used as a condiment with seafood dishes.

thyme A minty, zesty herb.

turmeric A spicy, pungent yellow root. It's the source of the yellow color in many mustards.

vegetable steamer A perforated insert designed to fit in or on a saucepan to hold food to be steamed above boiling water.

vinaigrette A light salad dressing made with oil, vinegar, and seasonings.

vinegar An acidic liquid often made from fermented grapes, apples, or rice and used as a dressing and seasoning.

wasabi A Japanese plant that tastes like strong horseradish and is used in a powder or paste form.

water chestnut A white, crunchy, juicy tuber popular in many Asian dishes.

whisk To rapidly mix, introducing air to the mixture.

white mushroom A button mushroom with an earthy smell and appealing soft crunch.

white vinegar Vinegar produced from grain.

wine vinegar Vinegar produced from red or white wine.

zest Small slivers of peel, usually from citrus fruit.

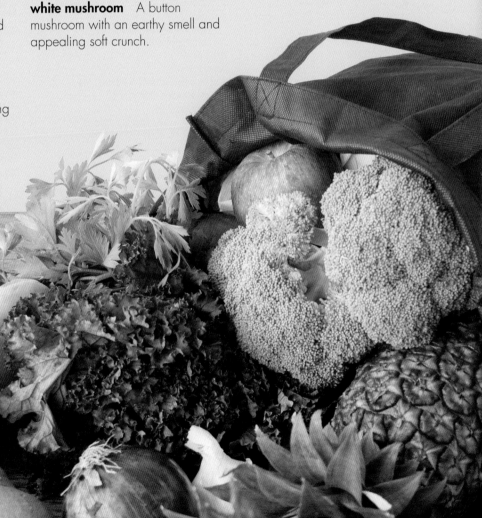

Index

All photography by Amari Thomsen, with the following exceptions:

p14 Andy Crawford © Dorling Kindersley
p14 Chris Villano © Dorling Kindersley
p14 David Murray © Dorling Kindersley
p15 David Murray and Jules Selmes
    © Dorling Kindersley
p17 © Masterfile

p19 Lorenzo Vecchia © Dorling Kindersley
p29 Sian Irvine © Dorling Kindersley
p29 Gaby Cheikh © Dorling Kindersley
p52 Dave King © Dorling Kindersley
p177 William Reavell © Dorling Kindersley
p214 Dave King © Dorling Kindersley

p215 Philip Dowell © Dorling Kindersley
p216 Lorenzo Vecchia © Dorling Kindersley
p217 Stuart West © Dorling Kindersley
p217 Will Heap © Dorling Kindersley
p218 Lorenzo Vecchia © Dorling Kindersley